Extreme Rapid Weight Loss Hypnosis
for Women

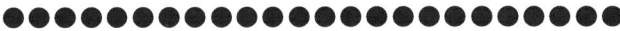

●●●●●●●●●●●●●●●●●●●●●●●●●●●●

**Natural and Rapid
Weight Loss Journey.
You'll Learn:**
Powerful Hypnosis • Psychology
Meditation • Motivation • Manifestation
Mini-Habits • Mindful Eating

Michelle Guise

contained within this document, including, but not limited to, errors, omissions, or inaccuracies.

Download the AUDIOBOOK VERSION of This Book for FREE

If you love listening to audiobooks on-the-go, I have great news for you.

You can download the audiobook version of this book for FREE just by signing up for a FREE 30-day Audible Trial! See below for more details!

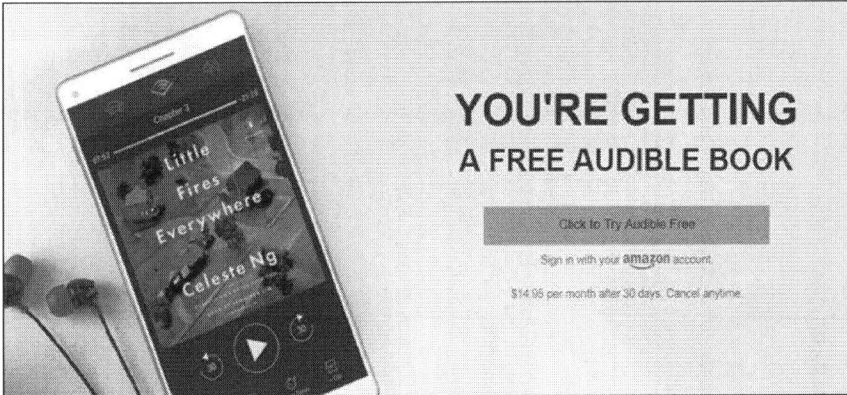

Audible Trial Benefits

As an audible customer, you will receive the below benefits with your 30 days free trial:

- FREE AUDIBLE COPY OF THIS BOOK

- After the trial, you'll get 1 credit each month to use on any audiobook

- Your credits automatically roll over to the next month if you don't use them

- Choosing from Audible's 200,000+ titles

- Download the free Audible app

- Listen anywhere with the Audible app across multiple devices

- Make easy, no-hassle exchanges of any audiobook you don't love

- Keep your audiobooks forever, even if you cancel your membership

- And much more...

Follow the QR Codes Below to GET STARTED!

For AUDIBLE US	For AUDIBLE UK

For AUDIBLE DE	For AUDIBLE FR

Table of Contents

Introduction

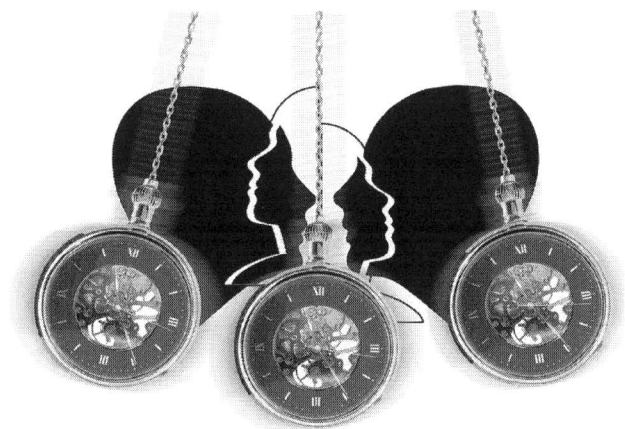

Figure 1: "Our life is shaped by our mind, for we become what we think"- By Bhudda

"I had to wear men's shoes because my fat would just drape over the ankles of ladies' footwear. I have always loved clothes and feeling feminine, so that was soul-destroying," recalled Dee Chan as she told the *Daily Mail* (Keegan, 2015). Dee weighed about 518 pounds (235 kilograms), a state which, according to her, made life miserable. She wouldn't go to just any restaurant; she had to be sure she could fit into their chairs first. Clothes in her size were difficult to come by, so she had to make her own using curtain fabric.

After many attempts at other options like fad diets and weight loss support groups to lose weight, Dee's hope was slowly getting out of reach. Dee finally came across Steve Miller, a clinical hypnotherapist and motivational trainer, which marked her dawn to a new day. She consistently committed herself to guided weight-loss hypnosis exercises, and three years down the line, Dee had lost 238 pounds (108 kilograms)! She was now weighing 280 pounds (127 kilograms) and still going down to her target of 168 pounds (76.2 kilograms).

Gaining weight can be a thorn in the flesh for women, especially with the rising concern to maintain body shapes. It could be that you were in the same boat with Dee, or you probably have gained a little more pounds but still feel uncomfortable with the new weight. Even using public transportation and sharing seats becomes difficult as other passengers are usually not comfortable sharing their space with you. You would probably understand, but the inner pain is unbearable as you admire others with less weight.

Apart from the emotional pain, weight gain is associated with various ailments that make life less enjoyable. One condition is obesity, which may, in turn, lead to cases of high blood pressure, coronary heart disease, type 2 diabetes, breakdown of cartilage and bone in joints, stroke, gallbladder diseases, or even death. Living with the fear that one day, these diseases may catch up with you is equally unbearable. It might be that you are already a victim of these diseases, and you feel that you want to fight it by dealing with the root cause, that is, weight gain.

You probably tried other options such as exercising, but still couldn't see the positive results. Could it be a case of slow metabolism, or did you find it hard to maintain consistency with your exercises? Slow metabolism is when the rate at which your body burns fewer calories is low, irrespective of whether you are at rest or active. In such cases, exercises are not so helpful. Additionally, hormonal birth control methods such as implants are reported to increase body weight (Okunola et al., 2019). Therefore, even after watching their diet and exercising, women may still find themselves gaining weight.

You may have tried many other tools for weight loss, but don't give up yet. Thomas Dexter Jakes once said, "When you're tired, it's a sign that you're almost at the end of your fight." Have you ever heard of or tried hypnosis? Hypnosis is a weight-loss tool, which is increasingly gaining acceptance due to the positive testimonies that its loyal users have. It is a natural method, which presents less negative effects than strict dieting and exercising. Apart from weight loss, hypnosis enhances positive behavior such as quitting smoking, promoting good sleeping habits, emotional stability, and eases anxiety. Therefore, by engaging in hypnosis as a weight-loss method, you could kill two birds with one stone.

This book will guide you through a natural and rapid route that makes weight loss a reality, mainly through hypnosis. You will also learn other important factors of weight loss, such as meditation, mindful eating, and other mini-habits that we usually take for granted. This book will equip you with the relevant knowledge that empowers you to practice hypnosis with confidence and purpose. Take the stride that will land you to your last stop in your endeavors to lose weight, by reading and practicing the contents of this book and earn your testimony. Don't deprive yourself of the best you, so let's get started. Let's begin by knowing each other.

Meet Michelle Guise

Michelle Guise is a former professional swimmer, teacher of oriental holistic disciplines, and an expert in psychology. With over 23 years of health and nutritional experience under her belt, she has dedicated her career to helping people of all ages lose weight naturally through alternative methods that pose no danger to health than most restrictive diets and exercise regimes. Michelle was initially motivated to study weight-loss methods by her older sister, whom she helped to lose 64 pounds (29 kilograms) in just a few months. Today, Michelle Guise promotes natural weight loss methods all over Europe and North America and has already helped numerous people shed extra pounds and regain their health without dieting and exercising. Michelle is, therefore pleased, to guide you through to losing those extra calories the hypnotic way.

Chapter 1:

Can Thoughts Reshape Your Body?

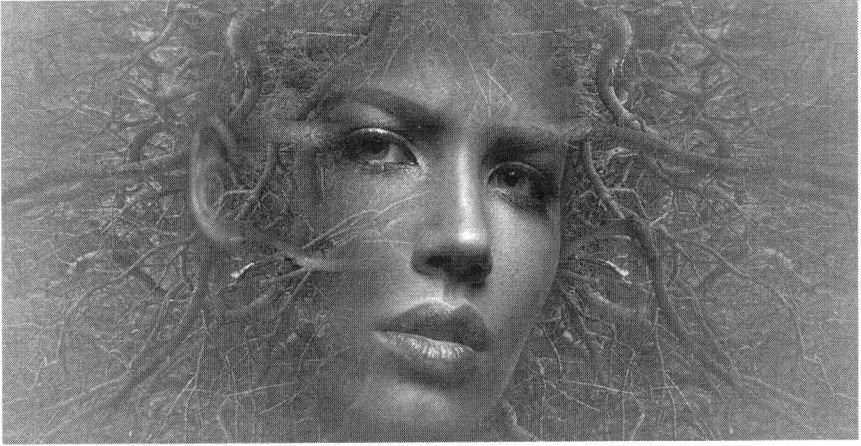

Figure 2: Thoughts can reshape your body.

Quite often, we tend to separate the mind from the body, yet the two interconnect and affect each other. When it comes to reshaping our bodies, our focus is usually on the body itself, but does the mind have no role to play in what happens to the body? Mariamme Williamson said, and I quote, "You must learn a new way to think before you can master a new way to be." Everything begins with your thoughts, and weight loss is not an exception. You are a product of your thoughts in all aspects of your life. Your thoughts could either be the culprit to pull you down or the hero to exalt you. You may blame your failures on the environment, workmates, spouses, or the government but often leave out the main culprit—your thoughts. Consciously appreciating and utilizing the interactions between your thoughts and body towards what you want to achieve is key. Once you learn how to tame your mind's thoughts, you learn to explore your better self, and surely, you can reach beyond the sky. This chapter will enlighten you on the role of thoughts in reshaping your body.

Why Diets Don't Work

You might have tried following strict routines for dieting and exercising before, or maybe you have yet to. If you subscribe to the latter, then this book just got you right before you experienced great frustrations. At first, it looks like it works but months or years down the line, you realize that you still gain more weight. While the principle of dieting and exercising seems to make sense, even scientifically, how come it doesn't seem to work? Various things contribute to the limited or short-lived success of diets, and we will explore these in this section.

The Principles of Dieting

The market is practically flooded with various types of diets and new fitness regimes that are always presented as the final stops in searching for effective weight loss methods. In some cases, diets are combined with exercising to increase the rate at which the weight loss takes place. To understand why diets do not work as expected, let's begin by looking at how diets are purported to work.

Diets are basically based on three principles as follows:

- **Some diets are based on limiting the intake of carbohydrates:** The body has a limit as to how much carbohydrates it uses for metabolic processes. In the body, carbohydrates break down into glucose, which is, in turn, taken up by cells in the body and used as energy to drive all body activities, including blood circulation and breathing. Excess glucose is usually converted into glycogen, which is stored in the liver. If there is still more excess glucose in the blood, it is stored in the form of fat as an energy source in cases of emergency. Therefore, dieting limiting consumption of carbohydrates assumes that when you limit the amount of carbohydrates that you take in, you increase the chances that all of them will be used up by the body and reduce the possibility of carbohydrate to fat conversion.

Starches, sugars, and fibers are all different types of carbohydrates. Starches are found in foods like pasta, rice, potatoes, bread, and cereal products. Foods that contain sucrose (table sugar), fructose (fruit sugar), and lactose (milk sugar) are rich in sugar carbohydrates (Mayo Clinic, 2020). Fiber is mainly found in plant-based foods such as vegetables, whole grains, and legumes, where they are known as roughage. Various diets depend on altering the amount of these carbohydrates. In most cases, starches and sugars are reduced, while fibers are recommended, mostly for their roughage.

Some of the ways carbohydrates are reduced in diets are: replacing sugars with sweeteners, raising fiber content instead of starchy foods, refraining from drinking fruit juices, cutting down on bread, and opting for low carbohydrate breakfast foods such as eggs (Spritzler, 2016).

- **Other diets are based on eating low-fat ingredients:** Extra fat in the body is stored inside specialized fat cells, which are called the adipose tissue (Harvard Health Publishing, 2019). As amounts of available fat in the body increase, the fat cells either expand or new cells are created to accommodate the extra fat. This results in an increase in overall body weight. Therefore, diets that encourage individuals to reduce fat ingredients aim to reduce the amount of body fat available for storage in the adipose tissue, thereby presumably trimming body weight.

Low-fat diets are foods where the amounts of calories attributed to fat are limited to 30% and below (Bhandari & Sapra, 2020). This implies that if a food provides 100 calories, it is only classified as a low-fat food if three grams or less come from fat. Dietary fat exists as monounsaturated, polyunsaturated, trans, and saturated fats. Their differences lie in physical and chemical properties. Essentially, monounsaturated and polyunsaturated fats are in the liquid form at room temperature, while trans and saturated fats exist as solids. However, by consuming one gram of either the liquid or solid fats, one consumes nine calories (Bhandari & Sapra, 2020). This amount of calories is high compared to the amounts consumed in a gram of carbohydrates or proteins.

Although all the types of fat add too many calories that enhance weight gain, low-fat diets are also developed with serious consideration of these types of fats. This is because trans and saturated fats are regarded as unhealthy since they raise low-density lipoprotein (LDL), which is the greater part of the body's cholesterol (CDC, 2020). Polyunsaturated and monounsaturated fats do not raise LDLs and are regarded as healthy and beneficial. Therefore, low-fat diets recommend larger amounts of the "liquid" fats, although the overall "30% and below" range should be maintained. E Between these "liquid" fats, it is suggested that monounsaturated fats should contribute up to 20%, while polyunsaturated fats contribute up to 10% of the total recommended fat calories in each food (Bhandari &Sapra, 2020). Low-fat diets recommend foods like vegetables, lentils, egg whites, fruits, whole-grain foods, legumes, chicken and turkey breasts without skin, white fish, and skimmed milk.

- **Diets that work in combination with exercises:** While some dieting programs are solo, some are designed to work hand in hand with exercises to enhance rapid loss of weight. The exercises could also be of one type, or they can be combinations of different types of exercises. Two major forms of exercise are often adopted, namely, cardio exercises and strength training.

Cardio or aerobic exercises, also known as endurance exercises, are rhythmic activities that raise the heart rate, increasing the body's metabolic rate. The increased metabolic rate implies that the body will burn out extra calories, even long after the exercise has been completed. This is the underlying principle for these exercises in aiding weight loss and body reshaping. They do not necessarily have to be lengthy as some reports show that even 10-minute daily sessions are effective if done consistently (Waehner, 2019). Examples of cardio exercises are cycling, running, jogging, brisk walking, and swimming.

Strength or resistance exercises involve working your muscles harder than they usually do, mainly by using your body weight or working against an external resistance. When an individual engages in strength activities, their muscles contract, and tiny tears appear on their muscles. The tears will gradually heal while the new muscle tissue appears to repair the muscles. By so doing, individuals attain a lean appearance, among other benefits such as a better aesthetic appearance. Lifting weights, gardening activities like digging, push-ups, squats, and climbing stairs, are examples of strength exercises.

What Then Goes Wrong?

From the information you have learned so far, you would agree that the principles that lie behind diets and exercises are logical and are supposed to work. How then is it that they end up not working? All of these dieting methods mentioned above have one thing in common; that is, they all focus on the body and its metabolic processes. They highly rely on the most common weight loss model based on the manipulation of calorie intake-consumption ratios. Simply said, diets are developed based on assumptions of how much calories they will release into the body and how much of those calories would be used during the body's metabolic processes. Essentially, an individual has to take in fewer calories than they will burn, so they ultimately lose weight. That makes sense, right? What then goes wrong? Diets may work for a limited period of time, but their efficacy is questionable in the long run. About 95% of the people who lose weight through a change of diets regain it or even more within a period between one to five years (Selig, 2010). In this section, I will explain why conventional diets do not work in the long run.

The body recognizes diets as stressors: When we change diets by, say, reducing carbohydrate and fat intake, with time, the body interprets the lower calorie levels in the body to be a stressor, and it responds accordingly. Normally, the body produces cortisol and adrenaline, both of which are stress hormones, to counter the "stressful conditions." In this case, the hormones reduce the rate at which the body consumes calories, partly by reducing the rate at which metabolic activities take place. This becomes a distraction to reducing weight, resulting in little to no weight loss and possible weight gain.

Diets are a "surface way" of approaching weight loss: Diets are usually approaches that are based on external instruction and reception of eating habits. The instruction is simple, "Stop eating that, but instead, eat this." That's all. It is like approaching a matter from the surface, not the root cause. What is it that causes individuals to prefer foods that are damaging to their bodies and, at the same time, adding to their weight? Most diets do not address that, which makes them appear like written rules that are just followed for the sake of it. They are not incorporated into the inner being of an individual, which is a step that would make the dieter endure for longer and yield better weight-loss results. Involving the inner being helps tap into the deep-rooted beliefs, patterns, and behaviors that play an important role in informing our choices of food and the reasons behind our preferences (*3 reasons why diets don't work*, 2018).

Diets are too constraining: Most diets often involve an inflexible restriction on what one should eat and what they should not. Most of such diets are not close to what an individual used to eat before the diet commenced. The only willpower that people have towards dieting is derived from the fact that they are desperate to lose weight. Otherwise, no pleasure is derived from the process. Diets, therefore, deprive people of enjoying the process of losing weight and becoming healthier. Additionally, the stress involved in coping with the new recommended diets leads to the production of stress hormones, which reduce the rate at which calories burn in the body. The ultimate effect is that the weight-loss process becomes hampered, and individuals may gain weight instead.

Diets can cause eating disorders: It has been reported that people who diet are presented with a risk of being victims of eating disorders, eight times more than those who do not diet (Selig, 2010). Individuals may find it easy to oblige to strict diets initially, but this may gradually become more difficult with time. As I have explained earlier, diets may slow down the rate of metabolic activities in the body. This could lead to starvation. Individuals may experience periods of extreme hunger, during which they are tempted to eat excessively. Consuming huge amounts of food within a short time, also known as binge eating, can be a supporting factor for weight gain.

Products touted as low-fat products: Since some diets are based on consuming low-fat foods, people scout for these products when they buy their food. They check if the food has the "low-fat content" tag or any information that shows that the food is low in fat. However, some manufacturing companies present products as "low-fat foods," yet they replace the fat with refined carbohydrates in huge amounts (Bhandari, 2020). Refined carbohydrates are low in fiber and are digested quickly. This causes surges of sugar levels in the blood, followed by excessive hunger as all the food is used up too quickly. This way, refined carbohydrates lead to overeating, making the intended weight loss impossible.

Diets often overlook other factors that cause weight gain: Food intake and consumption is just a part of the causes of weight gain. Other factors are involved, and if the weight gain is due to such factors and are not addressed, individuals continue to gain weight even after committing to consistent dieting procedures. Other factors that cause weight gain include health conditions and medications, age, hereditary genetics, sex, environment, lack of sleep, and emotional factors such as stress.

The Psychology of Eating

If focusing on our carbohydrate and fat intake, bodily functions, and metabolism is not the answer to permanent loss of weight, then what is? How about involving the mind in the equation? For almost a decade now, considerable effort has been made to establish a connection between one's mind and weight loss. This collaboration between the mind and the body falls under the discipline called the psychology of eating. Psychology of eating explores behavioral, nutritional, and physiological aspects that explain why, what, and how we eat (Harvard University, n.d.). In other words, the discipline examines "eating behavior," without only focusing on physiological and nutritional factors, but the whole being, including the mind. Although your main goal is to lose weight, understanding the psychology of eating and positively altering your perceptions towards eating has extra benefits. These include improved alertness, increased body flexibility, and a more positive relationship with food (Cleveland Clinic, 2016).

Factors Affecting Food Choices

Choosing what to eat was not much of a difficult task thousands of years ago, as it is now, especially in western and westernized regions of the globe. This was probably because there wasn't much variety back then, which would impair people's choices on what to eat. Nowadays, there is a ***greater abundance and variety of food***, which is relatively ***cheaper***, a state which makes food choices very difficult to make. Such abundance and variety also, to some extent, encourage unorganized, impulse, and binge eating, all of which are push-factors toward gaining weight. Normally, when the energy levels in the body have been diminished, signals are sent to the brain to alert it on the need for food, and the brain triggers ***hunger***. In response to hunger, we consume food, and when we are satisfied, signals are sent to the brain again to stop the eating (Meule & Vögele, 2013). However, sometimes, the balanced control of food consumption by the brain is overridden by people, triggered by the abundant food availability.

It has been reported that there is a natural connection which links eating with *moods and emotions*. Food choices are highly triggered by a variety of emotions and moods. For example, food choices differ when one is sad, happy, celebrating, or depressed because food is often used to cope with or reinforce emotions. It is normal that humans eat to survive, which is in response to hunger, but there are cases when we eat, not to satisfy the hunger motive, but as a response to emotions. For example, some prefer to drink alcohol when they are angry because they believe that the drink would calm them down. On the other hand, alcohol can contribute to weight gain because it is packed with sugar, carbohydrates, and empty calories (The Recovery Village, 2020). We can use our emotions to determine and monitor when, what, and how we eat. If we can control our emotions, we can equally control our eating behavior to make it healthier.

Choices of food and consumption patterns can be influenced by external factors, such as *advertising and packaging*, leading to impulse buying and eating. These factors can be better controlled by training the mind to make conscious choices that promote healthy eating; otherwise, gaining weight would be inevitable. Please note that healthy eating does not only imply being aware of the quality and quantity of nutrients that you consume but also enjoying eating as an activity.

Other factors that influence our choices concerning food are:

- **Family:** The food preferences of family members can also influence your individual choices about food because it is easier to prepare meals that everyone will eat and enjoy than to make separate meals for members of the same family.
- **Economic status:** Some studies show that the costs of food are dependent on the quality and safety of the food. In that regard, low-income families are financially disadvantaged and cannot afford better quality food, and so, they resort to cheaper foods that are often unhealthy (Lo et al., 2009).

- **Social:** Friends influence food choices and eating habits. If you go out with your friends, the likelihood of eating similar foods is high despite your differences.
- **Genetics:** Results from one study reported that a variant of the genes for bitter taste receptors determines whether an individual enjoys drinking coffee or not (Nutrition, 2018). Therefore, genetics can affect the food choices of individuals.
- **Cultural:** Perceptions of foods differ from cultures. Some cultures strictly exclude some foods from their diets, say, pork or all meats.

Weight Management Through The Psychology of Eating

Through extensive research, some researchers have discovered groundbreaking insights into how to use the mind to lose weight permanently. Psychology refers to the study of the human mind with a special focus on particular behaviors. This means that psychology explores how people do what they do and the reasons and motivation for their actions. In weight loss endeavors, psychology can be applied in two ways. First, psychology can be used to deal with **behavior**. In this case, an individual's eating patterns are identified, analyzed, and used to determine relevant changes in eating behaviors. Any factors that influence the eating patterns of an individual are also explored. Second, psychology can focus on **cognition**. The way we think affects our eating patterns. For example, self-defeating patterns of thinking are often associated with limited willpower in making relevant efforts to manage weight. The psychology that is focused on cognition is more effective because it addresses both thinking and behavioral patterns concerning eating.

Cognitive therapy explores your thoughts towards food, as this determines your eating patterns. It involves various aspects, which, if done appropriately, could aid effective and permanent weight loss. The first thing that you should do is **set your goals**. For example, you could say, "I want to lose 35 kg of weight." With your goals in place, you need to realize that the journey may not be easy, but you need to **develop the willpower** that will drive you towards realizing your dream. Since time immemorial, one of the things that human beings fear is change. To make weight loss a reality, **be ready for change**, be it in the way you think, behave, eat, shop, or even relationships. **Learn to monitor yourself** and discover what causes you to eat at any given moment. This helps you determine the alterations you need to make in your eating patterns and adjust accordingly. Such adjustments could be on the size of your food portions, types of foods, or how often you consume food.

Breaking linkages is another important aspect. This involves altering or coping with conditions that would normally trigger you to overeat. For example, don't store unhealthy foods in your refrigerator because as long as they are available, you are compelled to eat them. The principle that you apply in breaking linkages is distractions, which involves replacing unhealthy lifestyles with healthier ones (Cleveland Clinic, 2016). You can as well replace negative and self-defeating thoughts with more positive coping ones. Self-defeating statements include:

- "For how long will I endure this? It's too hard."
- "I can't wait to start eating my goodies again, as soon as I reach my weight target."
- "If it doesn't work within the next year, I will call it quits."
- "The last time that I tried to lose weight, it didn't work. This might not work as well."

When you accommodate such thoughts in your mind, you are either accepting failure or creating it. Besides, you make the weight loss process less enjoyed. Better results are expected when you enjoy every step of the way. You should create a positive mindset through positive statements like the following:

- "What really triggered me into overeating? I need to identify what it is so that I put in place countermeasures should I encounter the same trigger again."

- "Maybe I should not keep ready-to-eat products in the house because as long as I see them, I am tempted to eat even when I am not hungry."
- "I must reach my target weight and maintain it."
- "My main goal is living a healthy lifestyle, and then I will lose weight in the process."

Thoughts and statements such as these are encouraging, and they add fascination to the whole process of losing weight. I like to call such statements "cheer statements" because they cheer you on in your weight management endeavors.

Evidence Supporting the Role of the Mind in Weight Loss

The involvement of the mind in weight management is not an idle philosophy. It is supported by results and conclusions from scientific research experiments. In this section, I will explore such evidence to exhibit the authenticity of the information concerning the link between the mind, body, and weight loss.

Dr. Linda Solbrig and Colleagues' Research

This study was done at the University of Plymouth, in the United Kingdom (UK). The study aimed to compare two motivational interventions to see which of them would be more effective in enhancing weight loss. The compared interventions were Motivational Interviewing (MI) and Functional Imagery Training (FIT). In the MI program, the person who desired to shed weight went through counselling sessions that guided them to precisely identify and voice what motivated them to achieve their lower weight targets. In the FIT program, the candidate for weight loss was taught to visualize themselves, achieving their goal of losing weight. They also learned to visualize themselves doing the things that they could not do due to their current weight, that they would be able to experience once they lost weight (Cohut, 2018).

Methods: The World Health Organization (WHO) stipulates that individuals with body mass indexes (BMI) of 25 are deemed as overweight, while those with BMIs of 30 are classified as possibly obese. Therefore, 141 participants whose BMIs were 25 and above were selected for the study, and 55 of them underwent MI, while 59 underwent FIT. Two sessions per individual were done for each intervention—a phone session and a face-to-face one. Follow-up calls were made to all the participants for six months, such that the total contact time for each participant was four hours for the whole study period. Assessments were done immediately after the completion of the study at six months, as well as 12 months after the study's completion.

Results: FIT participants lost 4.3 cm more from their waists over six months than the MI participants. Participants in the FIT group lost an average of 4.11 kilograms, while those in the MI group lost 0.74 kilograms. The FIT group further lost 6.44 kilograms after the 12 month-extension, while the MI group lost 0.67 kilograms. In general, FIT participants lost five times more weight, on average, compared to the MI participants.

Conclusion and takeaways: The FIT intervention was effective in shedding the weight of the participants. It is interesting to note that the participants were not restricted to any form of diet or exercise regime. They were free to make their own choices on food and lifestyle, while the researchers supported their choices. This study proves that the participation of the mind is a tool for effective and rapid weight loss without adhering to a stipulated diet. Gradual or abrupt loss of motivation is usually one of the factors that make most efforts to lose weight to fail. In this study, FIT helped the participants to maintain their motivation throughout the study and long after its completion. The key principle in the efficacy of FIT was the mindshift that gave the participants the zeal to be what they visualized about themselves, and that became their source of motivation.

Eric Robinson and Colleagues' Research

It is reported that distraction, awareness, memory, and attention are cognitive processes that impact food intake patterns. This review study's main objective was to analyze whether these cognitive processes affect the amount of food taken by individuals (Robinson et al., 2013). Information on the effects of these cognitive aspects on food intake can be used to deduce the effects of mindful or attentive eating on food consumption. This gives light on whether the mind has a positive role to play in aiding weight loss.

Methods: The studies that were selected to be part of this study were original researches, whose methods were based on manipulating the attention of individuals before eating or modifying memories of formerly eaten food, before observing the effects on food consumption. Twenty-four studies that matched the review's inclusion criteria were used to conclude this review study.

Results: The information from the selected research suggested that distractions while eating resulted in an average increase in the immediate consumption of food but greatly decreased distractions in subsequent meals. Whenever the memory of the consumed food was enhanced, lower later intake of food was observed. When visual data on the amount of food that was consumed during a meal was removed, this raised the immediate intake of food by individuals. Enhancing the awareness of the eaten food did not have any effects on immediate intake.

Conclusion and takeaways: It was concluded from this study that attentive eating does have a role to play in determining food consumption. This also implies that attentive eating could influence the loss of weight in people. Therefore, it was suggested from the study that attentive eating be incorporated into other interventions that are aimed at aiding weight loss.

Coordination of Eating by the Human Brain

We have extensively explored the connection between eating food and the brain at a psychological level. However, there is a connection between these two at a physical level too. Since the brain is responsible for controlling all processes that take place in the human body, it certainly needs vast amounts of nutrients. It is not just any nutrients, but quality nutrients that promote the brain's efficiency (Calvo-Ochoa & Arias, 2019). Interestingly, the brain also controls the eating process and other processes that are involved in making nutrients available.

If five people were to be given the same plate with the same type of food, their perceptions and thoughts concerning the food would be different. For example, a person who is trying to lose weight may see the food in view of how much fat and sugars it has, and essentially, how many calories they may get after eating. These may not be the same thoughts for an athlete, scientist, or any other person. The different thoughts and perceptions that we have towards food determine how the brain will respond when we eat (David, n.d.). In this section, I will delve into the specificities of what actually happens in the brain when you eat. As the saying goes, "Knowledge is power," enlightenment on how our choices of foods physically affect the brain, and ultimately other parts of the body, motivates us towards mindful eating.

When you eat, your mind communicates with the digestive organs through the brain, spinal cord, and nerves. Even before you eat food, the image of the food you want to eat is pictured in the cerebral cortex, a part of the brain where functions such as sensations, perceptions, and thoughts about anything, are processed. The processed information about the food is then sent to the part of the brain called the limbic system through nerve impulses. Emotions and physiological functions like hunger, blood pressure, thirst, and heart rate are regulated in the limbic system. All the sensory, emotional, and thought information about the food, as conveyed from the cerebral cortex, is processed in the hypothalamus, which is a small collection of tissues found within the limbic system. The hypothalamus converts this information into physiological processes in the body (David, n.d.).

Suppose you are eating a chicken drumstick, and it's your favorite part of a chicken. It is more likely that you are going to enjoy the eating process. This information will be coded as I have described earlier. When it reaches the hypothalamus, this organ will modulate this positive input by sending activation signals through the parasympathetic fibers, to parts of the digestive system, namely, salivary gland, gullet, stomach, intestines, pancreas, liver, and gallbladder. Once digestion is initiated, your food will be broken down, absorbed, and assimilated more efficiently. You will also burn calories more effectively.

If for any reason you do not like to eat the chicken drumstick or feel guilty about eating it but still eat it, the hypothalamus will receive this negative information input. It will respond by sending signals through the sympathetic fibers of the central nervous system. This action stimulates inhibitory responses in organs that are part of the digestive system. This implies that your food will not be efficiently digested and will probably stay much longer in the digestive system. The burning of calories will be too slow and inefficient due to the release of hormones such as cortisol (David, n.d.). By the way, the mind cannot differentiate between imagined and real stressors, so stress hormones like cortisol are released to cope with both cases. All these aspects suggest that the food will be converted to fat for storage, a process that supports weight gain.

Chapter 2:

What Exactly Is Hypnosis?

Various medical and therapeutic benefits have been derived from the application of hypnosis, especially in the fields of pain and anxiety (Klein, 2014; Solomon, 2012). One of the most recent applications of hypnosis within the past few years has been its use in enhancing weight loss. However, many misconceptions surrounding the concept of hypnosis make the true understanding of what hypnosis is appear blurred. In this chapter, you will achieve a clear understanding of what hypnosis is, how it works, and the different types that exist.

What Is Hypnosis?

Hypnosis is a mental state of reduced consciousness during which an individual does not respond to external stimuli, and no voluntary action is involved. This state partly resembles sleep, increases focused attention, reduces external awareness, and enhances elevated suggestibility (Psychology Today, n.d.).

Hypnosis and Sleep

Disturbed and insufficient sleep are some of the effects of major diseases such as hypertension, obesity, cardiovascular disease, and Alzheimer's disease. Interestingly, hypnosis can enhance deeper sleep in individuals who have insomnia. Moreover, sleep-walking is closely analogous to what is witnessed in a person who responds well to hypnosis ("Sleep and Hypnosis," 1934). It can be typically difficult to clearly identify whether an individual is sleeping or hypnotizing from a single glance. Even with such a resemblance between sleep and hypnosis, there are notable differences that separate the two. Such differences include the following:

- During hypnosis, an individual is in their best state of awareness, which is not the case with sleep.
- During sleep, body muscles are relaxed, while they are rigid during hypnosis ("Sleep and Hypnosis," 1934).
- When an individual falls into a sleep, even a light one, they are not responsive to any suggestions. People in deep hypnosis are readily obedient to suggestions.
- Knee-jerks are less pronounced or absent in sleep, while they remain unreduced in hypnosis.

Hypnotic Induction

How does a hypnotist guide their client into a state of hypnosis? It all boils down to hypnotic induction, which refers to the process of establishing a set of conditions that create a hypnotic trance. Hypnotic induction is the foundation for the success of any type of hypnosis. When their clients enter hypnosis, hypnotherapists use "state deepeners" to ensure that the clients are fully hypnotized and maintain the ability to respond to suggestions during the hypnosis procedures (Hypnotc, 2019). Let's explore the various ways through which hypnotic induction is done.

There is one step that is usually general to all types of hypnotic induction. In all forms of induction, the hypnotist should **build rapport** with their client as this enhances healthy communication. This is done by creating a sense of connectedness and commonalities between themselves and their clients. The effect of this strategy is that the client will tend to trust the hypnotist more because they will feel that they are well understood. Generally, because people tend to like themselves, they are more likely to like and trust other people who share some similarities with them. The trust that is built this way makes it easier for the client to enter into a hypnosis state.

The most common hypnotic induction technique is called **progressive relaxation induction**. As the name suggests, this technique involves a gradual transition into hypnosis, which utilized various components to enhance the process. To begin the hypnotic induction, the hypnotist gives various suggestions to the client and encourages them to follow the instructions. Various suggestions can be made during progressive relaxation induction. Some examples are given below:

- *Muscular relaxation:* Here, the focus is on various body muscles. The client should reach a state where they are well-dipped into what they would have been instructed to do, taking note of all the sensations involved. For example, the hypnotist could say, "Focus on your upper body, and allow it to relax. Relax your body parts as I mention them: chest, stomach, shoulders, arms, and neck. Completely relax them now." As the hypnotist calmly makes the suggestions, the client is taken through a journey that explores the different parts of their upper body, gradually shutting the stimuli from the external environment away.

- *Visualization:* This method takes the client into an imaginary world. Our bodies respond to imaginary situations in the same way they would to real situations because the mind cannot distinguish between the two. Therefore, the imaginary relaxation that the client is guided into by the hypnotist has soothing effects on the body, helping the client enter a state of hypnosis. To use visualization as a tool for hypnotic induction, the hypnotist could say, "Imagine a beautiful, wonderful, peaceful, and relaxing place. Now imagine you are in that place, absorbing the wonderfulness in it. Take heed of how relaxed you are feeling as you explore the relaxing environment in the place you see in your mind..." The client will adopt the relaxed state and be susceptible to hypnotizing.

- *Breathing:* In this case, the client is guided to focus on breathing patterns to shift their focus from the environment and begin to be hypnotized. This could involve systematic breathing patterns or simple inhale-exhale breathing. The suggestion could be, "Inhale. Keep inhaling. Take note of the feeling of your lungs that are full of air. Now, slowly release the air by breathing it out. Take note of how relaxing that is." When the client successfully acquaints themself with the relaxing state of exhaling, they become more ready to be hypnotized.

- *Counting:* This is a more cognitive approach to inducing hypnosis. The hypnotherapist could use suggestions like, "When I count to a certain number, you can allow yourself to go deeper into this state of hypnosis. Let's start with 10…" (Hypnotc, 2019).

The response of the clients to the induction procedures depends on their preferences. For example, some would prefer physical suggestions such as breathing and relaxing their muscles, while others better accept analytic approaches like counting. Some may even find it easier to engage with visual suggestions. Progressive induction is more successful when the instructions are given in a manner that is easy to follow.

Rapid hypnotic induction is another option for guiding clients into hypnosis. Unlike progressive induction, rapid induction is quick and less time-consuming. It is more relevant in cases where the hypnotist has to cut down the induction time to increase the time for the actual therapy. It can also be used when the client is in pain. Three forms of rapid induction exist as follows:

- *Shock inductions:* This refers to psychological, not electric shock. Here is why psychological shock can be a powerful tool to enhance hypnosis. Every now and then, we go through shock and surprise. I am sure you are also familiar with the feeling of these two emotions. Each time we are shocked or surprised, we undergo instant and profound hypnosis. Hypnotherapists distract their clients and introduce shock when they use it in inducing hypnotherapy. The shock will take the client by surprise, and while they are still in that state, the hypnotist will immediately suggest that their client should "sleep." As a way of dealing with the shock, the client would rather "sleep" than wake up and deal with the "fight and flight" response to shock.

- *Confusion inductions:* These work in the same way as shock inductions, with the only difference being that confusion inductions are based on confusing the client. This is done by overloading the client's head with simultaneous tasks that are extremely difficult to complete. For example, the hypnotherapist could suggest that the client should count backward from 10,000 in skips of 37 while moving their hand in opposite directions and singing their answers to the tune of the "happy birthday" song. You have probably felt the confusion upon reading this, right? That is the sole purpose of the suggestion. While the client is still confused, the hypnotist tells them to "sleep." So, the client would prefer to "hypnotize" than complete such a head-swirling task.

- *Pattern interruption induction:* In this case, normal subconscious patterns such as handshakes are interrupted, causing confusion in the client. While the client is still trying to come to terms with what is happening, the hypnotist tells them to "sleep," and they immediately enter into the hypnotic trance.

Eye fixation is another form of hypnotic induction. The hypnotherapist asks the client to fix their gaze on something, say, a light in the ceiling. The principle behind this hypnotic induction is that when the client faithfully gazes at one particular thing, their eyes will get tired. Once this happens, the hypnotherapist will suggest that the client closes their eyes, and by doing so, they go into a hypnotic state.

All the other methods of hypnotic induction that we discussed earlier are direct. However, hypnotherapists can employ an indirect method for inducing hypnosis, which is called **conversational hypnotic induction**. In this case, the hypnotist engages the client with a conversation that may or may not involve hypnosis topics. However, the talk should incorporate some hypnosis-inducing suggestions embedded within the conversation. While conversational induction can be used on its own, some hypnotists prefer to use it at the beginning of other types of hypnotic inductions to prepare their clients for deep relaxation during hypnosis. Conversational inductions may include statements like, "It's wonderful to note that *you are already relaxing*, even though we sat down just now," or "We wouldn't want you to *hop into hypnosis* a bit too soon, not until you are ready to *go into hypnosis*" (Hypnotc, 2019).

The Hypnotic State

Having understood how the hypnotic state is induced, you might then wonder how it feels like being in a hypnotic state. The way an individual feels when they are in the hypnotic state is similar to what they feel when they are meditating. You will feel relaxed and extremely focused. Physically, you may feel heaviness and relaxation in body muscles like the eyelids, almost the same way you feel when you are sleepy. Additionally, you may also experience slower, steadier, and shallower breathing, a tingling sensation in your fingers, and time distortion as time seems to move slower or faster. Your alertness to the environment becomes reduced as you go into a trance-like state.

What is the involvement of the brain when a person is in a hypnotic state? The brain consists of two cerebral hemispheres, that is, the left and right hemispheres. The left brain is dominant when one is awake, and it represents the conscious mind. The conscious mind deals with our intellect and verbal communication. The moment we relax or become hyper-focused on certain activities, the right hemisphere takes control. This side of the brain represents the unconscious mind and is more involved with our emotions and creativity (Williamson, 2019). Therefore, when one is in a hypnotic state, the conscious mind (left hemisphere) is bypassed, as the unconscious mind (right hemisphere) dominates. In this state, an individual can deal with their emotions more effectively and learn to control them.

The Fear of Being Hypnotized

Although hypnosis has been used for centuries, many myths and misconceptions surround the concept. Such misconceptions create a great fear of being hypnotized to many people, as they are not sure about what could happen, especially during their time in the hypnotic state. You could be one of such people, and this section clarifies issues around myths and misconceptions about hypnosis so that you hypnotize with understanding.

Can you be hypnotized to do things against your will?: One of the fears that emerge from the misconceptions about hypnosis is whether people can be hypnotized to do things without their consent. Such myths are usually based on, say, films where someone was probably turned into a zombie or a killing machine against their will (Watts n.d.).

As I explained earlier, hypnosis is not like sleep, where you could be unconscious of your external environment and what is happening to you. During hypnosis, you know what is happening to you. What makes you hear and follow the suggestions given by a hypnotist is that you are aware of their presence. When you follow the suggestions, you know what you are doing. With that being said, you have the right to refuse suggestions that you are given if they clash with your beliefs, integrity, or rights as a human being. So, the simple answer to the question is that you cannot be hypnotized against your will unless you let it.

Can you reveal personal secrets during hypnosis?: It is misconceived that when you are in a hypnotic state, your mind is always programmed to tell the truth, so you end up giving up your personal secrets and information during the process. This is not true. Some even suggest that you are more capable of telling better and more creative lies because of the access that you would have to unconscious resources (Watts, 2020). One can tell lies in a hypnotic state in the same way that they would in their wide-awake state.

Can you get stuck in a trance forever?: There is a misconception that you can go too far in your trance, to the extent that you will not be able to come back to reality. Hypnosis is not a spiritual journey or incarnation; it is a state that we all go through every day as we focus on our daily activities. There have never been cases when one would be said to have been in a trance forever. If the suggestions by the practitioner do not wake a client up, they will simply wake up on their own or fall into a regular sleep, after which they will still wake up. In other words, one can simply open their eyes and reconnect to the external environment whenever they decide to wake up, even in the middle of hypnosis.

Here is the scientific explanation for this. The electroencephalogram (EEG) measures brain waves of different frequencies in the brain to determine brain activity, which is also associated with physical activity. Raw EEG is usually described in terms of frequency bands as follows: Gamma (greater than 30Hz) Beta (13-30Hz), Alpha (8-12 Hz), Theta (4-8 Hz), and Delta (less than 4 Hz) (Neurohealth, 2019). When brain activity is highest, the brain waves are in the Gamma range. During hypnosis, brainwaves are either in the Alpha or Theta ranges, both of which are associated with slow physical activity and high relaxation. The highest level of relaxation happens when brain waves are in the Delta range, in which state one falls into a deep sleep and then wakes up.

Does hypnosis contradict religious beliefs?: Generally, hypnosis is not representative of any of the various religions that exist around the globe. There are indeed some religions and churches that restricted their members from subscribing to hypnosis sessions. However, in modern-day, the ethical use of hypnosis is being supported by various religious sects, as it helps people overcome problems such as pain, phobias, and addiction. Churches such as the Roman Catholic and Orthodox and Hinduism, Buddhism, and Judaism are some of such religious groups (hypnosisalliance.com, n.d.). If there are any concerns about religious beliefs, the client should open up to the professional hypnotist so that the hypnotist's suggestions would not go against the client's faith.

Are there people who cannot be hypnotized?: Some myths suggest that there are people who cannot be hypnotized. As long as an individual can sleep and wake up, they can be hypnotized because hypnosis is a natural process. Consider how we sometimes get sucked in movies, to the extent that we see the movie as though it's taking place in real life. Remember that moment when you suddenly come back to your "senses," and you get surprised that you had been shedding tears because of a movie. That's a state of hypnosis that most of us have probably gone through. As long as we can go through such moments of extreme focus, we can go through the hypnosis as guided by a hypnotist, on our own. However, the extent to which every individual is susceptible to planned hypnosis is different. About 10% are highly susceptible to hypnosis, while 60 to 70 percent are moderately hypnotizable (Wilkinson, 2020). The rest may find it difficult to enter a hypnotic state, but they eventually do.

Some even suggest that intelligent people cannot be hypnotized. Intelligent people naturally have an elevated sense of focus, creativity, and imagination. Research reports that intelligent people get into a hypnotic state more easily than individuals whose intelligence is below average (Harris, 2016).

How Does Hypnosis Work

During hypnosis, a trained hypnotist or hypnotherapist induces a state of heightened concentration or focused attention. This process is guided through verbal cues, which are referred to as suggestions. Repetition is key, as it emphasizes and reinforces the instructions that are given by the hypnotist. Other skills, such as changing tones in speech, can make suggestions even more powerful.

All our emotions, thoughts, and cravings begin in the unconscious part of the brain. The conscious part of the brain then responds and acts according to the information coded by the unconscious mind. As I explained earlier, during hypnosis, the unconscious mind is dominant. Therefore, one can explore their unconscious mind during hypnosis, which enables them to reframe their unconscious urges.

All types of hypnosis typically follow certain steps. However, there are steps that are general to all types of hypnosis, and these are:

1. **Induction into hypnosis:** We have extensively explored various types of hypnotic induction and highlighted that hypnotic induction involves everything that is done to aid your transition from your wide awake self to your hypnotized self. Everything that is done to enhance the switch from using the highly conscious mind to using the unconscious mind is part of the hypnotic induction process.

    A professional hypnotist can induce hypnosis in a face-to-face encounter, or people can use recordings or memorized scripts. Whichever the case might be, the first thing is to make oneself comfortable. This could be done by sitting on a comfortable chair or lying on a comfortable couch or bed. Since hypnotic induction also requires the exclusion of external stimuli as much as possible, your eyes need to be closed. While in this position, various hypnotic induction methods such as controlled breathing techniques, muscular relaxation, visualization, and counting can help you to relax and focus.

2. **The state of hypnosis:** This is when you would have entered the hypnotic state. This state is characterized by an elevated state of relaxation, focus, and alertness, as I have alluded to earlier.

3. **Suggestions:** Hypnotic suggestions are statements that are meant to alter the state of thoughts of the subconscious mind by replacing unwanted thoughts and upgrading outdated ones. They can also be used to deepen the state of hypnosis. They are based on the principle that humans depend much on communication, and meanings of words can provoke responses that emanate from the mind. Once suggestions have been made during the hypnotic state, they remain effective in the mind for at least a day to several weeks (Watts, 2020a).

There are different ways with which suggestions are made. The most common and traditional way is the direct form of suggesting, where ***direct commands*** are made. The commands should emphasize the preferred outcomes, and they should be clear. For example, the hypnotist could say, "You eat when you are hungry," or "You eat to survive, not for the sake of it." That way, the unconscious mind is reprogrammed to, say, trim down or even stop binge eating. Due to its authoritative nature, direct suggestions' efficacy could depend on factors such as life experiences and an individual's upbringing. People who are not used to taking orders might find it difficult to accept direct commands during hypnosis.

Sometimes, less authoritative forms of suggestions are used, and these are called ***indirect commands***. Such suggestions range from simple indirect statements to metaphorical ones. An example of a simple indirect suggestion is, "You *might* be already feeling intense relaxation throughout your body." While the hypnotist may seem like they are not sure of what their client is feeling, they are suggesting that the client should "feel the relaxation throughout their body." On the other hand, metaphors are statements with a related meaning, which is not literal, but they sometimes convey the message better than the direct statement. For example, "It's time to climb to the top of the mountain" could mean that it's time to make your success a reality, but the former exerts more emphasis than the latter.

Alternatively, **neuro-linguistic programming (NLP)** uses suggestions that closely resemble the way we think. NLP depends on the fact that every individual has their own real "selves" based on their environment, behaviors, capabilities and skills, beliefs and values, identity, purpose, and spirituality (Skills You Need, n.d.). Changes in any of the factors can affect changes in other factors. For instance, a person tends to overeat when they are in an *environment* where food is abundant and eat less when there is little to no food available. In this example, *behavior* has been affected by the *environment*. Here is an example of how NLP can be used: *"Imagine an image of a body shape that you do not like, say, an obese image. Concentrate on how it makes you feel. Then imagine the image gradually becoming smaller and turning into black and white. See it moving away from you until it eventually disappears. Take note of the feeling that this gives to you. Now, imagine an image of the body shape that you desire. Make the picture grow bigger and bigger in your imagination. Again, note how this makes you feel."*

Understanding the laws that govern hypnotic suggestions is of paramount importance, as these provide some seemingly simple but powerful tricks that make the suggestion achieve their purpose. Let's have a look at these laws (John Mongiovi, n.d.):

- **Law of Reversed Effect:** This law is based on the fact that the resistance that arises when one tries to do something increases with their efforts. It's a "the more you try, the harder it becomes" kind of situation. Therefore, this law suggests that the focus should not be on "avoiding fats or sugars" because focusing on this is, by interpretation, means focusing on resistance. Rather, the focus should be on the desired outcome.

- *Law of Dominant Effect:* Naturally, individuals tend to remember emotional events more than neutral ones. Therefore, attaching emotions to suggestions makes them more memorable. The effects of emotional suggestions are stronger when one is in a hypnotic state, where emotionality and suggestibility are higher.
- *Law of Concentrated Attention:* Repeatedly focusing your attention on an idea or situation tends to enhance its reality. This law applies even in negative situations where the problems people face are due to their concentrated attention on the causes of the problems. In much the same way, when one concentrates their attention on desired outcomes, the outcome tends to realize itself.

4. Awakening: When the required duration of hypnosis is over, the hypnotist will gradually guide their client through a process of awakening and reconnecting with the external environment and reality. The transitions have to be gradual to make it as natural as possible.

Types of Hypnosis

Now that you have a clear understanding of the steps involved in hypnosis, I will take you through different types of hypnosis. Before then, I would like to clear the misunderstanding that comes with "hypnosis" and "hypnotherapy." These two words are often used interchangeably but are they the same thing? Hypnotherapy is a form of guided hypnosis that is done with a professional clinical hypnotherapist (Psychology Today, n.d.). Simply said, hypnotherapy is a branch of hypnosis. Having clarified this, let's explore the different types of hypnosis. There are two types of hypnosis: guided hypnosis and self-hypnosis.

Guided Hypnosis

When most people talk about hypnosis, they mean guided hypnosis because there is a tendency to think that hypnosis always has to be guided by someone. This is a misconception. Guided hypnosis is one of the two types of hypnosis, and it exists in three forms.

Hypnosis guided by the hypnotherapist in person: In this case, an individual has a one-on-one encounter with a professional hypnotherapist. The advantage of this type of guided hypnosis is that the whole process is customized. There is no "one size fits all" approach to hypnosis in this case. The hypnotherapist can design the procedures, duration, and suggestions according to a client's requirements to ensure that they achieve their goals.

Hypnosis guided by a hypnotherapist in absentia: In this case, hypnosis is also guided by a hypnotherapist, but not in a face-to-face scenario. In this case, the instructions and suggestions can be found in the form of audios, which are often available online. One simply has to download these and listen to them, following the instructions just as they would in the physical presence of a hypnotherapist.

Hypnosis guided by the client: The client records themselves on a smartphone or any other type of recorder, giving instructions and suggestions for a hypnosis session. They will then use this for their own hypnosis session. They could either use their own words entirely or read scripts written by a hypnotherapist. Others would prefer to leave a space at the beginning of their recordings to give themselves time for induction so that the recording would catch up with them when they have entered the hypnotic state. However, if one prefers this type of hypnosis, it is recommended that they learn how to induce hypnosis properly and structure autosuggestion (Di Napoli, 2019). This will give you the confidence to guide your own hypnosis successfully.

Self-Hypnosis

Also known as unguided hypnosis, self-hypnosis is when you become engrossed in a hypnotic experience while you give yourself positive suggestions that enhance the realization of your goals. Hypnotherapists are not involved in this case, which makes it an individual encounter. This practice helps you have upgraded control over your thoughts as all the suggestions are self-created and align with exactly what you want to achieve (Harley, 2020). However, the hypnotic procedure is more or less the same as guided hypnosis. You will get to understand more about self-hypnosis in the next chapter.

Chapter 3:

Self-Hypnosis for Weight Loss

In her testimony, Emily Farris described how she tried different weight loss tools with profound frustration until hypnosis became her final stop. She tried two juice cleanses, seven half-hearted rounds of Weight Watchers, marathons, different types of crash diets, and weight loss pills. Emily admits that she would lose a few pounds here and there but would still gain more than she would have lost. She said, "Slowly, those extra 15 pounds that I 'd never been able to shake turned into an extra 20, and then an extra 25." She was beginning to give up and had the support of family, friends, and even doctors who thought she had tried enough. The day Emily decided to try hypnosis marked her own end to a dark tunnel (Farris, 2016).

Were you on the verge of giving up on your desire to lose weight? You probably have tried different forms of dieting and exercise regimes, all of which might have worked, but not for long. Don't give up yet, at least not until you try hypnosis as a tool for losing weight. Since the 90s, there have been reports from various studies that suggested that people who coupled dieting with hypnosis lost weight at least twice more than those who just dieted without involving any cognitive therapy (Lefave, 2019). Not only does hypnosis enhance rapid loss of weight, but it also helps to maintain your desired weight for longer. This chapter explains how hypnosis can be used as a weight-loss tool and presents self-hypnosis in more detail.

How It Works

Hypnosis is not a magic bullet that will help you shed weight in seconds or within a day. As established in Chapter 1, the key to rapid and permanent weight loss lies in changing your eating habits and training your brain to make healthy choices, and this requires some time. Self-hypnosis helps you break unhealthy patterns in food choices and frequency of eating, thereby reprogramming your mind to make better and healthier choices when it comes to food.

Self-Hypnosis Modifies Behavior

Hypnosis works by addressing the observable behavioral patterns that promote weight gain. It is often used as a tool for making behavioral modifications and habit corrections. We adopt behaviors and habits as a factor of time, and some of them end up becoming part of the characteristics that define us.

Behaviors are programmed in the subconscious mind in response to suggestions that are made through the five senses: touch, sight, hearing, smell, and taste. Here are some of the ways through which behaviors are programmed in the subconscious mind (Grimes, 2015):

- Past experiences
- Identification with the traits of parents or peers
- Acceptance of ideas that are brought forward by authorities
- Repeated exposure to a situation
- Hypnosis

Hypnosis maximizes on the fact that if behaviors can be learned, they can also be unlearned and replaced by other behaviors. When you enter the hypnotic state, your subconscious mind is dominant, and therefore, you have direct access to the part of the brain which programs your behaviors. The hypnotic state presents a heightened state of learning, during which you are highly susceptible to suggestions that are meant to modify and update your behavior (Wilkinson, 2020). The suggestions that are made are directly deposited into the subconscious mind, bypassing the conscious mind, which tends to reason a lot. This way, behaviors are modified.

Let's say the bad behavior is binging, frequently responding to cravings for fats and sugars, as well as a lack of activity or exercise. These are there, programmed in your subconscious mind. When you are hypnotized, the suggestions that are made erases these unwanted and unhealthy behaviors from the subconscious mind, without the resistance from the conscious mind. These suggestions also program the desired, healthier behaviors that support the right choices of foods and the patterns of eating and exercising. Unlike stipulated diets and exercises which may not provoke interest in individuals, hypnosis promotes the joy and zeal in putting the healthy choices to practice. As we alluded to earlier, food that we eat with joy and acceptance is digested and metabolized better than what we eat with disgruntlement.

The reason why it is difficult to modify behaviors while you are awake is because the conscious mind will be dominant. The conscious mind has a memory factor, which remembers any previous efforts that would have been made to change behaviors and reverse them. At the end of the day, no behavioral changes are witnessed. This concept is referred to as the "critical factor" or "criticizing factor" of the conscious mind (Serenity Hypnosis, 2013).

The Conscious and Unconscious Mind

Now that you know that behaviors are modified in the unconscious mind, let us explore the conscious and unconscious mind more to fully understand how the two influence changes in behavior during hypnosis. To begin, let's differentiate between the conscious and unconscious mind.

The conscious mind is the one that is dominantly active during the day as we go about our activities. It is also referred to as the "thinker" because it governs contemplation, logic and reasoning, deliberations, judgments, and acceptance. The conscious mind occupies the left side of the brain, a space that amounts to 10% of the whole brain (Grimes, 2015). On the other hand, the unconscious mind is on the right side of the brain, and it occupies 90% of the whole brain. This part of the brain is the one that is active when we are relaxed and inactive, such as when we are sleeping. It is referred to as the "doer," and its functionalities include governing pain avoidance, habits and beliefs, pleasure enhancement, feelings and memories, and the autonomic nervous system.

The autonomic nervous system is the part of the nervous system that supplies all internal organs of the body, without the conscious effort of an individual. Therefore, it regulates the bodily functions that are controlled by those various organs, and these include digestion, metabolism, heart rate, excretion, respiration rate, pupillary response, and sexual arousal. The autonomic nervous system is composed of the sympathetic and parasympathetic nervous system, which are antagonistic to each other.

The ***sympathetic nervous system*** (SNS) controls emergency and stressful situations in the body. It does this with the help of spinal nerves that connect internal organs to the brain. When a stressful situation is detected in the body, the spinal nerves are stimulated. The body is prepared for the stress by increasing the heart rate, dilating airways to make breathing easier, increasing blood flow to the muscles, releasing stored energy, decreasing blood flow to the skin, and increased sweating. In such stressful times, the SNS decelerates processes such as digestion.

By controlling metabolism, the SNS controls weight loss or gaining weight. The SNS controls daily energy expenditure by regulating the resting metabolic rate, and initiating thermogenesis in response to stimuli such as changing energy states, food intake, and carbohydrate and fat consumption (Thorp & Schlaich, 2015). The activation of the sympathetic nerves that supply the liver, skeletal muscle, adipose tissue, and pancreas enhances catabolic responses such as glycogenolysis and lipolysis. Lower lipolysis leads to future weight gain (Nishizawa & Shinomura, 2018). Additionally, since hypnosis modifies behavior, it makes eating healthy food more enjoyable than stressful. This increases the efficiency of the metabolism of the food.

Unlike the SNS, the ***parasynthetic nervous system*** (PNS) controls the functions of the internal organs during normal situations. It primarily consists of the vagus nerve and the lumbar spinal nerves and usually plays conservatory and restoration roles. The parasympathetic division reduces heartbeat, blood pressure, and breathing rate while it stimulates digestion and waste elimination. Interestingly, research that was done by Costa and colleagues reported that when diets and exercises are done for weight loss, the parasympathetic activity is increased, while sympathetic activity is reduced. The opposite was reported to be true for weight gain (Costa et al., 2019).

The Role of Emotions in Behavior

The conscious and unconscious mind work together to modify bad behaviors into desired ones. The motivation to stop a behavior is developed in the conscious mind that makes decisions based on rational information. For example, it is decided in the conscious mind to say, "I will stop eating too much animal fat because it is hazardous to my health and can lead to obesity." The subconscious mind will then act upon the decision that would have been made in the conscious mind, and then it manifests in the physical as behaviors and habits. In other words, suggestions are planned logically using the conscious mind, and we then use them during hypnosis to reprogram the unconscious mind.

When you binge eat, the decision would have been made in the conscious mind and then implemented by the subconscious mind. To change a bad behavior that has been recognized by the subconscious mind for a long time, you need to change the decisions and motivation in the conscious mind. What happens is that the subconscious mind responds to the stronger emotion from the conscious mind. There are always two emotions in the conscious mind, but one is stronger than the other. For instance, when one decides to overeat, they also think about not overeating, but that is overpowered by the desire to overeat.

Therefore, to successfully change behaviors, the desires in the conscious mind should be modified so that the subconscious mind can pick new suggestions.

For example, say, binge eating is the unwanted behavior. The first thing would be to weaken the emotion or motivation that is associated with the behavior. This could be, "I will eat as long as the food is available. What's the point of not eating when the food is there?" The conscious mind should adopt another motivation, which supports a new behavior. This could be, "I know I used to eat for the sake of it, but I now need to take care of myself and adopt healthy patterns of eating." Whenever the zeal to binge eating comes, you emphasize the new decision, thereby making the emotions that are associated with the unhealthy behavior progressively weaker while empowering those associated with healthier behavior. The subconscious mind will pick the stronger emotion and exhibit the behavior that is associated with it. Attaching strong emotions to the behaviors that we prefer makes them more susceptible to being adopted by the subconscious mind.

Therefore, if you attach strong emotions to behaviors that promote weight loss, they become reprogrammed in the subconscious mind, become part of you, and you exhibit the behaviors more naturally. This does not happen instantly. The old and undesired behaviors will often come through. They will only permanently shut away when you persistently continue to give power to the new behavior so that it becomes your new norm. The Law of the Dominant Effect comes to play in this case.

How Hypnosis Targets the Subconscious Mind

Think of your subconscious mind as a Global Positioning System (GPS) that will guide you towards the "destination" you have given it. The subconscious mind is active when the body is in a more relaxed state. In that state, the subconscious mind accepts suggestions better. That is where hypnosis comes in. It enhances a heightened state of relaxation, thereby providing the subconscious mind with a conducive environment for it to perform as desired. While in that state, suggestions are deposited directly to the subconscious mind, where they gradually push away negative behaviors and replace them with desired ones.

I introduced the concept of brain waves in Chapter 2. In this section, I will further explain the association of hypnosis with this concept. In the Beta state, you are fully awake, and the subconscious mind has zero contribution to what would be happening. When you are in the Alpha state, you are dominantly conscious but sometimes fall into moments of subconsciousness when, for example, you are dipped in a TV series, driving long distances, or daydreaming. In the Theta state, you are dominantly subconscious and slightly conscious. You are fully subconscious when you are in the Delta state. What all this information means is that hypnosis takes place when the mind is the Alpha and Theta states, where it is possible to swing between the conscious and unconscious states. One you move from these states, you either end up being in the Beta state, where you are fully awake, or in the Delta state, where you are deeply asleep. This also further clarifies the concerns about one going too far in hypnosis. You can go no further than the Beta and Delta states.

Is Weight Loss Hypnosis Viable?

Coupling weight loss plans such as diet, exercise, and counselling with hypnosis can help you lose some pounds faster and for longer too. However, the application of hypnosis in weight loss is relatively new, considering that it only attained extensive research attention in the past decade, and there is still limited information on the effectiveness of the method. A few studies have made efforts to analyze the efficacy of hypnosis in aiding weight loss.

There are many factors that determine the viability of weight loss hypnosis. These include:

- **The number of hypnosis sessions:** In one study, the effects of hypnosis on weight loss were analyzed on 31 obese women whose ages were between 21 and 71. It was concluded that the more hypnosis sessions, the greater the weight loss (Clarke, 2019).

- **The suggestions that are used:** A study done by Deyoub and Wikie (1980) observed the effects of hypnotic suggestions compared to task motivation and control groups on weight loss. Their results showed that hypnotic suggestions were more effective because remarkable weight loss was observed in the group that had received suggestions. However, the type of suggestions is as important as the way they are presented, as both factors affect the efficacy of hypnosis. Essentially, suggestions that are meant for weight loss should be specific so that they address the matter. Unspecific suggestions may show less efficacy.

- **For how long does it work?:** The efficacy of hypnosis in weight loss is addressed as a factor of immediate weight loss and the long term stretch. This is where most complaints about various techniques that are used for weight loss come from. Weight loss is witnessed in the first few months, but individuals tend to gain more weight in the long run. Hypnosis enhances long term weight loss because the behaviors that promote weight loss are programmed in the subconscious mind. In one study, it was reported that the weight loss that had been achieved through hypnosis could be maintained even after two years (Clarke, 2019).

- **Hypnotizability:** Like we discussed earlier, all people can be hypnotized, but the extent to which we are all hypnotizable differs. There is a positive correlation between hypnotizability and weight loss. The study that was done by Andersen (1985) led to the conclusion that people who are highly hypnotizable tend to achieve hypnosis-induced weight loss at a faster rate than those whose hypnotizability is either moderate or low.

- **The depth of the hypnotic state:** Even among highly hypnotizable individuals, the depth of the trance differs. However, some studies support the notion that the deeper the trance, the greater the weight loss. The opposite was also reported to be true (Jupp et al., 1986).

Further Evidence on the Efficacy of Hypnosis for Loss of Weight

In this section, I present some of the studies that were done that show that weight loss hypnosis is viable.

Hypnotherapy works as a treatment for obesity (Bundrant, n.d.): In this study, 60 women who qualified as obese were categorized into three groups: one who received hypnosis together with audiotapes, another who received hypnosis only, and the control group. Observations and evaluations were done after one and six months from the commencement of the experiments. The results that were observed showed that there was significant difference between the groups that received the treatment compared to the control group. However, the two groups that received hypnotherapy showed no significant difference between themselves. The research concluded that hypnotherapy is an effective treatment for diabetes. Considering that weight gain is one of the common symptoms of diabetes, the fact that hypnotherapy can treat diabetes implies that it can also treat the weight gain that accompanies it.

Hypnosis alters brain connectivity (Faymonville et al., 2003): In this study, the aim was to analyze any alterations in cerebral functional connectivity associated with the hypnotic state than the resting state and simple distractions. Positron emission tomography (PET) scans were used. The study involved 19 highly hypnotizable and right-handed participants who were exposed to hot noxious or warm non-noxious stimulation of the right hand during mental imagery, resting state, and hypnotic state. Brain areas that showed a response to noxious stimulation under the modulatory action of the midcingulate cortex only in the hypnotic state were identified. The results showed that the 50% reduced pain perception was attributed to hypnosis, as compared to the resting state. There was no significant difference in pain perception between the mental imagery and rest state. It was concluded from the study that hypnosis increased the connectivity in the midcingulate cortex and a large neural network that is involved in pain regulation. From these studies, we also deduce that if hypnosis can alter and improve connectivity in the brain, it is effective as a weight loss tool as it can alter physiological processes in the body.

Self-Hypnosis Methods

Taking yourself into a hypnotic trance is nothing like those scenes of stage hypnosis in movies. Through your imagination, you can create virtual experiences and powerful "memories" that help you believe and accept that you already achieved your weight-loss goal. In the previous chapter, we discussed a lot about hypnosis, which is guided by professional hypnotists. In this section, you will learn various methods for hypnotizing yourself, but before we delve into that, I will discuss the steps you should follow for successful self-hypnosis.

Steps to Perform Self-Hypnosis for Weight Loss

Through some research, scientists have proven that self-hypnosis can be done to lose weight. One of the powerful techniques of self-hypnosis is *visualization*. Here are the steps that make self-hypnosis through visualization work:

- **Breathing deeply and relaxing:** It is best that you schedule your self-hypnosis session for the early mornings when you are still drowsy or immediately before you go to bed when you feel sleepy. Choose an uninterrupted space where you can either sit or lie down. You can customize the place to your liking to make it even more relaxing. You can consider putting on soft music, using some essential oils to create pleasurable aromas, or burn incense. Specifically, identify your target amount of weight and the period you want to achieve it and say it aloud before you begin hypnosis. Be sure to say this positively. When you are ready, begin by rolling your eyeballs as if you are staring at the ceiling, or your hairline. Begin to inhale and exhale slowly and concentrate on your inhale-exhale patterns. This is how you will prepare your mind to get into hypnosis.

Now, imagine yourself in a beautiful, calm, and peaceful place. This could be a place close to a waterfall, with the peaceful, whooshing sound of the water. It could be a beach or any other place of your choice that makes you feel relaxed. Wherever you choose to be, make your experience there as enjoyable as possible. Allow all your senses to be part of the whole experience, smell the pleasant odors, see the views that are pleasant to the eyes, and hear the pleasant sounds around the place. Let all your senses be fully embedded in the experience.

- **Picture your desired body shape:** You need to program your mind with the body shape and size you want to achieve. Remind yourself about the amount of weight you want to shed off. Picture your targeted shape in your mind and view yourself putting on the dress you have always desired, that your current shape wouldn't let you wear. Envision people showering you with compliments of how awesome you look, and take note of the pleasant sensations that this triggers in you. Imagine the happiness, peace, lightness, and confidence that your new shape will bring. Be as precise as possible as you state what you want, and your brain will capture that.
- **Change perceptions through positive suggestions:** Successful self-hypnosis involves modifying negative perceptions into positive ones. While you are in a hypnotic state, you need to get rid of thoughts like, "I will always gain more weight" or, "Losing weight is difficult." If you entertain

them, your mind will accept and act on them. Rather, shift your focus to your desired results and feed your mind with positive suggestions like, "From now on, I choose to eat healthy food when my body needs it," or "My body now enjoys exercising. Besides being fun, exercising makes me feel strong and confident." Keep repeating such positive affirmations to your inner mind until they become part of you. Always be sure to attach the feelings you want to experience once you have achieved your goal of losing weight. This will serve as a motivation that will keep your mind focused on the goal.

- **Reorient yourself:** Now that your hypnotizing session is over, it's time to reconnect to external stimuli. To make the reconnection a gradual transition, count from 1 to 5 and make sure that by the time that you reach 5, you would have fully reoriented yourself. Use your senses to positively acquaint yourself with your environment by taking note of the pleasant aromas, the music, the orderly settings, as well as the confidence and peace that you feel. Be sure to take the internal experience you have had with you as you get off your chair, couch, or bed.

- **Repeat to perfect:** One hypnosis session is not enough to make you lose the weight you want. You need to regularly schedule more sessions to reinforce the suggestions that support your goal to lose weight while you get rid of negative thoughts and suggestions. As you keep emphasizing positive suggestions through repeated hypnosis sessions, your mind will become programmed towards those suggestions; you will find it easy to behave in ways that support your weight loss dreams. You will gradually find pleasure in following your exercising routines, let alone practice healthy eating. Your determination and positive attitude towards weight loss will grow with each session.

Other Self-Hypnosis Methods

Other variations exist to the hypnosis steps that I described earlier in this chapter. These variations could be in the induction phase of the hypnosis or the actual hypnosis. The variations in the actual hypnosis are usually in the suggestions made and the approach taken in making the suggestions. The method that I described in the previous section uses suggestions that are memorized. You could consider the following variations in the way you present suggestions to your mind during hypnosis:

- Download a self-hypnosis audio that has suggestions that match what you want and play them during your session.
- Make your own customized audio that presents what you want, the way you want it.

The biggest variations in self-hypnosis methods are in the way hypnosis is induced. To many, this part is the most difficult as many distractions can hinder its success and the whole hypnotic session—the more successful the induction, the better the hypnosis encounter. In the previous section, we used breathing as the hypnosis induction technique. Here are more induction methods that may enhance the success of your hypnosis:

Magnetic hands: This method should help you shift from your thoughts and concentrate on feeling the energy between your hands.

- Rub your hands together until you feel the heat.
- Pull your hands apart until there is an approximate distance of 4 inches between them.
- Begin to repeatedly move your hands slightly in and out and feel the natural magnetic pull between your hands. Be attentive to the sensations as they gradually grow stronger.
- When you begin to feel that your hands want to come together, close your eyes and begin to deepen your induced trance.

Natural sounds: You can play audios of natural sounds such as the sounds of birds, ocean waves, waterfalls, gentle rain, or crickets at night. These constant relaxing sounds will occupy your mind and help you to get into a hypnotic state.

The 3-2-1 technique: This technique is based on going through the things you see, hear, or feel in three cycles. Besides redirecting your focus from your thoughts, it also improves your visualization techniques.

- Identify three things that you can see. These could be anything—the walls of the room, sun rays coming through the window, a pen that fell on the floor, flowers in a vase, or a portrait on the wall.
- Then identify three things that you can hear. This could be the sound of music in the background, a cat meowing, the wind, or your own breathing sounds.
- Finally, identify three things that you can feel. For example, you can notice how your clothes feel on your skin, the weight of your earrings on your ears, the warmth in the room, or the cool breeze coming through an open window.
- Remember you have to repeat the cycle three times, so it's time to start the new round. However, in the second round, you have to identify two instead of three things you see, hear, or feel. These could be the same as you have mentioned before or different ones.
- On the last round, focus on one thing that you can see, hear, or feel.
- You will repeat all the steps mentioned above, with the only difference being that your eyes will be closed this time, so you will be identifying things that you see, hear, or feel in your mind. Imagination plays a crucial role at this stage.
- By the time you complete the final cycle while your eyes are closed, you will have entered the hypnotic state.

More Tips

While you go through your self-hypnosis session, there are essential tips that apply to any method of hypnosis you chose to employ, thereby elevating the chances of success. Some highlights are below.

- **Make your suggestions specific and realistic:** There is no point in making suggestions that are unrealistic because they are, in fact, unachievable. For example, the amount of weight you intend to lose should be realistic for the time period you would have set. Also, avoid making suggestions that have ambiguous meanings. It is best that you write your suggestions down to keep yourself focused and avoid even slight shifts from your goals.

- **Set your hypnosis goals:** Your weight loss goals should be clearly stated to aid more focus to your hypnosis session. How much weight do you intend to lose? In how much time do you intend to do this? What are the strategies that you have put in place to make this a success? What is the motivation that you have for achieving your goals?

- **Visualize your goals:** Visualization is a powerful tool in hypnosis and can be used alongside any other methods. Imagining your goals motivates you to make the necessary steps and behavior modifications for them to become a reality.

- **Create a self-hypnosis script:** A self-hypnosis script describes the whole process of your hypnosis session, from the point of induction to the moment of reorienting. It is written in a specific and procedural way to ensure a connected flow in all steps. The suggestions should be specific, instructive, and coupled with emphasis. A self-hypnosis script helps you to customize your sessions to meet your needs and goals.

- **Use positive suggestions:** Positive suggestions are one of the pillars in hypnosis because they pose as the motivation towards your weight loss journey. Here are some of the ways through which you can use positive suggestions: using encouraging statements to boost confidence, visualizing yourself meeting your weight loss goals, making statements that fend off fear, rehearsing healthy eating, and using phrases that positively reframe your eating habits and exercise patterns.

Gastric Band Hypnotherapy

Gastric band hypnotherapy is based on tricking the mind into believing that you have a gastric band fitted around your stomach. A physical gastric band goes around the upper part of the stomach, where it reduces the amount of food that one consumes, eventually leading to a loss of weight. Since the gastric band in hypnotherapy is only imaginable, only the positive effects of using it are obtained while the side-effects are nonexistent. Unlike the physical gastric band, gastric band hypnotherapy is virtual and does not require surgery.

Remember a good movie that you last watched. Imagine how you felt so embedded in the movie, to the extent that you seemed to have forgotten that it was only a movie and the people involved were only acting. You even got so emotionally involved and probably felt excited, sad, angry, or jealous. Somehow, your mind got so involved that it couldn't recognize that it was just a movie and responded in a way it would if the scene was real. This is the same concept underlying the use of gastric band hypnotherapy. There will not be a physical band, but your mind will believe there is and respond the same way it would if a physical band was on your stomach.

How It Works

Gastric band hypnotherapy is usually done with a hypnotherapist's help to enhance the feeling that someone is doing the surgery, making the mind believe it more. In that case, the hypnotherapist will begin by explaining to you what will happen during the surgery. For example, they will explain how they will make an incision on the stomach, insert the band, and make the closing stitches. They may also use aromas to make the surgery more authentic to the mind.

Like any other method of hypnosis, you will begin with relaxation techniques that help you to enter the hypnotic state. Therefore, you can choose to use any hypnotic induction technique of your choice. Once you enter the hypnotic state, suggestions are made to the subconscious mind. In this case, the suggestions are that you have a gastric band fitted on your stomach. The suggestion is repeated again to emphasize the presence of a precaution, which is meant to aid weight loss.

When you wake up, your post-hypnotic suggestions should tally with the hypnotic suggestions. For example, you need to continue to remind yourself that you have a gastric band and that you need to maintain it well to reduce the chances of its side-effects. That way, you will gradually notice that you will begin to eat less because your subconscious mind would have been programmed to accept that you have a gastric band.

Chapter 4:

Meditate the Weight Way

Meditation is a tradition that dates back to centuries ago but has recently gained popularity all over the globe. Meditation helps you be more conscious of your thoughts, including those that involve food preferences and consumption frequencies, and perceptions about exercising. In precisely the same way that meditation can help us with stress, sleeping, and focus, it can also impact our eating habits, thereby helping us manage our weight. Some research has reported that meditation can be used to address eating disorders such as binge eating and emotional eating (Horton, n.d.). In this chapter, you will learn about meditation as a tool for weight loss.

What Is Meditation?

Although various religions incorporate meditation in their teachings, meditation is less about faith but is a tool for enhancing awareness, peace, compassion, and consciousness (Bertone, 2020). By definition, meditation is a mental exercise that trains the mind to relax, focus, and be aware by focusing on the present moment (Live and Dare, n.d.). In the same way that physical exercise trains the body, so does meditation to the mind. With meditation, we are better able to tame our thoughts and redirect them towards positivity. However, it is not a fight with our thoughts, a training to observe our thoughts without a sense of judgment or feeling guilty. At the same time, meditation does not let the thoughts wander.

There are three aspects that define meditation, and these are:

- **Observation:** In this case, you focus on anything that would be predominating the present moment without necessarily gluing your focus on one thing. In other words, the focus continues to shift as the meditation experience progresses.
- **Concentration:** This involves giving undivided attention to one thing, which could be located either in the external or internal environment.
- **Awareness:** This involves remaining alert and undistracted.

To better understand what meditation is, let us look at different types of meditation.

Mindfulness Meditation

Mindfulness meditation is one of the most popular forms of meditation, and its origins are in Buddhist teachings. It involves paying attention to your thoughts, observing them, and learning not to judge them. All you do is let your thoughts pass through your mind the normal way they usually do. The difference is that in those other times, you usually don't take note of your thoughts, and if you do, you are often judgmental, as opposed to what mindful meditation then teaches you to practice. Many times, our minds tend to wander, even when we are trying to focus on something. During mindfulness meditation, you quickly learn to notice that your mind has gone to different places. You learn to acknowledge your present experiences without feeling overwhelmed, an art that gives you control over your emotions and thoughts.

Here are some steps that you can follow in performing mindfulness meditation:

1. **Schedule your session and prepare:** You need to set aside the time for mindfulness meditation. Also, decide where you are going to do it. This could be in your house, your garden, or any other space that you choose. Both the time and the space you choose should present little to no distractions because the

meditation needs you to focus. You can do it any time of the day, as long as it does not affect your focus. For example, in very hot regions, an afternoon meditation may not be very successful because people tend to be sleepy in such conditions.

2. **Choose a posture:** You can sit on a chair, bench, cushion, or rug and make sure that your back is straight. Some would prefer to close their eyes, but it's a matter of choice.

3. **Observe the present moment:** Begin to focus on what is happening in the present moment. Take note of all the sensations that you are experiencing in your body and concentrate on them. Be aware of your breathing patterns and how they make you feel. Alternatively, you can scan your body with your mind, from your head to your toes. Again, be sure to take note of all the involved sensations as you explore each part of the body. The goal of this activity is not to quiet the mind but to concentrate on what is happening in the "here and now" moment.

4. **Notice distractions and judgments:** You are more likely to note that your mind will once-in-a-while wander from the present moment. You may find yourself regretting something that you feel you didn't do right or worrying about what you will make for dinner. It is intuitive that you would feel like rebuking your thoughts, but calm down, notice the distractions, and refrain from making any judgments. Just let the thoughts pass through and continue to focus on the present moment. Mindfulness meditation is the act of returning to the present moment, not once or twice, but many times.

5. Wrap up: If you were closing your eyes, open them once the session is over and gradually reconnect to the external environment.

Spiritual Meditation

Sometimes life experiences deter us from understanding ourselves, and we end up living in pretense, to the extent of accepting even what we really do not want. Spiritual meditation helps you explore who you really are and connect with God or the universe, depending on your beliefs. Christians take meditation as a form of worship by reading the Bible and reflecting on their lives to align with the Bible's messages. Spiritual meditation can be done at home or at buildings of worship.

Depending on the type of faith that individuals subscribe to, some prefer to kneel, sit, stand, or lie prostrate as they perform spiritual meditation. Sometimes essential oils such as myrrh, sandalwood, frankincense, cedar, palo santo, and sage are used to heighten the meditation experience (Bertone, 2020). Some also burn incense during spiritual meditation to spiritually connect to God and send their prayers to Him.

Focused Meditation

Focused meditation involves staying in the present moment by focusing your attention on one thing, whether internal or external. You could focus on things like your breath, smells, sounds, tastes, or staring at a burning candle., Focused meditation is based on using any of your five senses to focus on something.

By reading the explanation about what focused meditation is, you could have said, "Just that?," because it sounds so easy. However, it is easier said than done, especially for beginners. Starting with a few minutes, which you can always upgrade as you get used to the art is recommended. Here are important steps to follow should you decide to do focused meditation (Scott, 2020):

1. **Choose what to focus on:** Most people find it easier to focus on breathing because many other types of meditation involve breathing patterns. However, you can choose anything else.

2. **Be comfortable and ready:** Find a comfortable sitting position. If you choose to sit on the floor, balance yourself with cushions to make sure that you are relaxed and your spinal cord is not bent. You can alternatively sit on a bench or chair, right at the edge, with your feet parallel to the floor.

3. **Relax:** Relax all parts of your body including your shoulders. In that relaxed position, begin to breathe from your belly.

4. **Focus on your chosen target:** Use your senses of smell, hearing, or sight to focus on your chosen focal point. The goal is to experience all the sensations that are involved as you focus on the focal point. Try not to think about it as this shifts your focus from the present moment.

5. **Control any diversions:** You may find yourself beginning to analyze the target or think about other things that happened or need to be done. If this happens, do not be hard on yourself. Rather refocus and continue with your meditation.

Movement Meditation

Some people find it difficult to sit down and focus on "still" meditation. Movement meditation is perfect for such people. Movement meditation involves slow movements through various positions, which are dome mindfully (Flarey, 2012). This type of meditation can be done while sitting or standing, as long as stillness is not part of the process. Walking is also a form of movement meditation, as long as it is done mindfully. This means that while you walk, for example, you should take note of all the sensations that you feel as you lift one leg and place it down as the feet touch the ground. Take note of the sensations in your hands and other parts of the body as you walk. If your mind wanders, as is usually the case, you can just tense a muscle or move a part of your body in a way that brings back attention to those parts.

You could try doing this movement meditation: stand up and lift one of your arms as if you are trying to get a fruit that is out of reach. Stand with your toes to make yourself taller. Explore the sensations that are involved in the arm that you have raised, as well as the toes. Bring the hand down and repeat the same procedure with the other hand.

Mantra Meditation

This type of meditation depends on the repetition of a mantra to clear the mind and focus on the present. A mantra can be a word, phrase, or sound and can be spoken quietly or audibly (Ramananda, 2007). After repeatedly chanting the mantra for some time, you attain deeper levels of awareness. Follow these steps as you do your mantra meditation:

1. **Choose your mantra:** Selecting your mantra may also depend on why you want to meditate to motivate you. Shorter phrases are preferable as they are easier to remember and repeat. Avoid words that stir bad memories because they will disturb your focus.
2. **Relax:** Sit on a chair, bench, or floor. Close your eyes and take a few deep breaths, after which you should let your breaths be more relaxed.
3. **Chant your mantra:** Audibly repeat your chosen mantra slowly and do this in unison with the natural rhythm of your breath. You can either chant half of the mantra as you breathe in and another half as you breathe out. Alternatively, you could complete the full mantra as you inhale and repeat it again as you exhale. After about 10 recitations, start saying the mantra quietly while you just move your lips. After another 10 recitations, say the mantra without moving your lips.
4. **Address wandering thoughts:** If your thoughts wander during the meditation, gently refocus on your mantra as you continue to repeat it quietly.
5. **End the meditation session** by taking a few breaths, sitting quietly for a minute or two, and noticing how you feel.

Transcendental Meditation

Transcendental meditation is an extension of mantra meditation. In mantra meditation, The only difference is that the mantra is a word, phrase, or sound, which usually has a meaning attached to it. In transcendental meditation, the mantra is a meaningless sound. Thoughts are allowed to come and go in transcendental meditation, just in the same way that you would watch a cloud pass by (Calucchia, 2019). The procedure for transcendental meditation is similar to that for mantra meditation, but you will use a sound typically learned from a transcendental meditation teacher as the mantra.

Progressive Relaxation

One of the responses that the body employs when you are stressed or anxious is muscle tension. Progressive relaxation, also known as the body scan, is a type of meditation that relaxes muscles. The procedure for progressive meditation is as follows (University of Michigan, 2011):

1. Breathe in and tense the muscles of, say, your hands and arms so that they are hard but not painful. Do this between 4 and 10 seconds.
2. Breathe out and relax the muscles in a sudden, not gradual manner.
3. Before you work on another set of muscles, rest for about 10 to 20 seconds.
4. Repeat the three steps described above for other sets of muscles, such as muscles in your hands and arms, neck and shoulders, buttocks, legs, feet, jaws, and forehead.
5. When you have finished relaxing all your muscles, count down from 5 to 1 before you reconnect to the present.

Loving-Kindness Meditation

Loving-kindness meditation is a self-care technique, which increases the capacity for connection, acceptance, kindness, forgiveness, and compassion towards oneself and others (Bertone, 2020; Scott, 2020). Receiving love and kindness are not easy things to do, and it's even harder to send them to others. This is one of the reasons why you need a lot of practice so that you can receive and send love with relatively greater ease.

There are three basic ways through which you can do loving-kindness meditation. You can do loving-kindness meditation to show yourself love, receive love from others, or give love to others. Therefore, I will explain how to do loving-kindness meditation in light of these three concepts.

In the meditation that you do to **show yourself love**, consider the following steps you can modify appropriately to suit your needs.

1. Make some time for your meditation and sit in a comfortable position. Ensure your back is straight and your feet are parallel to the ground if you are sitting on a chair. Gently close your eyes, take about five deep breaths, and let your whole body relax.

2. Begin to imagine yourself being in your healthiest state, both emotionally and physically. See yourself crowned with inner peace. Admire yourself and appreciate the person that you are. Fall in love with everything that defines you and enjoy the feeling. Now, direct more focus on your inner peace and begin to take relaxed breaths. As you do so, imagine that you are breathing out tension, unforgiveness, hatred, or dissatisfaction while you breathe in feelings of love, appreciation, satisfaction, and peace.

3. Recite four positive phrases that reassure you about what you have imagined for yourself. You could say, *"May I have inner peace and joy," "May happiness be part of me," "May I appreciate who I*

am, and who I will be," and *"May I be emotionally and physically healthy and strong."* Feel the warmth from the love that you are showering yourself with.

4. When you have finished your meditation, open your eyes, and reconnect to the environment around you. Be sure to revisit the experience that you have had during your meditation any other time so that you live it in that real-life space.

In the previous example, you were receiving love from yourself, but you also need to learn to **receive love from others**. You could learn this by following a few steps that are described below.

1. While your eyes are closed, identify a close relative, friend, or colleague who loves you. Begin to imagine that person standing on your right-hand side, sending love to you through wishes of better health, happiness, peace, safety, and excellence. Bask in the warm love that the person is showering you with.

2. Now, imagine the same person or another person that loves you on your left-hand side. See them sending you love as in the previous step. Imagine yourself taking in the love that they are sending to you.

3. Now, create another view in your mind where all your loved ones and friends are surrounding you, sending showers of blessing and love to you. Imagine the abundance of health, peace, love, and joy coming to you as they continue to wish you good. Receive it and feel the warmth that they bring.

Now, it's time for you to send love to someone else, apart from yourself. This art requires an understanding that you and other people are similar in one thing—that you all wish to be happy. Here are some steps that you can follow in learning to send love to others:

1. Re-imagine one of the people that you love standing to your right. Begin to send them the love that you feel for them. Shower them with warm wishes. You could silently say to

them, *"May your life be filled with joy, peace, and happiness. May you not experience pain and sadness. May you find fulfillment in your efforts."* Repeat these phrases four times.

2. Now, begin to imagine someone whose relationship with you is not more than just being colleagues, with no particular feelings attached. Repeat the phrases that you used above to send them love and warm wishes. Derive some joy and warm feelings in sending love to others.

3. Expand your focus, and imagine the whole globe in the form of a small ball. Bring yourself to the awareness that all the living beings on the globe crave to be loved. Begin to shower them with love and warm wishes as you have done previously with your loved ones and your colleagues.

4. Take two deep breaths, and notice how you feel after the experience. When you are ready to terminate your session, open your eyes.

Visualization Meditation

Visualization meditation is a meditation technique on its own though it is sometimes used together with other meditation techniques to enhance better focus on the experience. The technique is based on visualizing positive scenes, events, or images to enhance relaxation, peace, and awareness (Bertone, 2020). For example, the techniques that we explained for loving-kindness meditation include visualization meditation. Visualization meditation also involves creating images of yourself succeeding in achieving goals, which are specific, measurable, assignable, realistic, and time-related. This betters your focus and motivates you to achieve your goals.

Considering that there are many variations for visualization meditation, I will provide you with a procedure for one of them.

1. Get yourself comfortable as you would before any other type of meditation.

2. Close your eyes and let your body relax. Also, slow down your breathing so that it becomes more relaxed.

3. Begin to visualize a beautiful place that you love; it doesn't matter whether you have been there or not. Allow your senses to make the visualization more realistic and engaging. For example, see blooming flowers, wavy waters, rocks with amazing shapes, hear the sounds of birds, moving water, or some music, feel the cool breeze on your skin, and smell the pleasant aroma from the flowers, air, and water.

4. See yourself moving towards the place and imagine the feeling that comes with being in the place. Go deeper into your vision.

5. As you continue to breathe, imagine the air you breathe out takes with it all the things you do not like, while the air you breathe in brings all your desires to you. Notice the sensations that this brings.

6. When you are satisfied with your meditation experience, you can open your eyes and reconnect with the environment around you. Carry the feelings that you experienced with you as you leave the meditation scene.

How Meditation Affects Weight Loss

Some experts support the notion that meditation has a crucial role to play in aiding the loss of weight. The better part is that meditation is not even a costly technique, and anyone can do it when and where they choose. Some can meditate for five minutes a day and still reap the benefits of meditation. However, experts recommend that 20 minutes is a workout period that produces the best results (Zielinski, 2020). Where is the connection between meditation and weight loss?

According to your desire, meditation causes the conscious and unconscious mind to work together in implementing alterations to your previous behaviors, (Zielinski, 2020). Such changes could be in your response to cravings for sugars, fats, and other unhealthy foods that promote weight gain. In the same way, meditation can also adjust your eating patterns. All behaviors, including those that promote weight gain, are found in the unconscious part of the mind. Therefore, if any changes in behavior should successfully take place, the unconscious mind must be included. As you meditate, you become aware of the behaviors that promote weight gain. That becomes the foundation for making the relevant changes to your behavior so that you can shed weight and maintain your desired weight.

The twenty-first century is highly characterized by busy schedules, as people search for means of survival. That alone is a huge source of stress. Stress hormones such as cortisol are released in stressful conditions, and these commands the body to convert calories into fat for storage. Therefore, it is difficult to lose weight as long as stress levels are high. This is where meditation comes in. Meditation has been proven to reduce stress and anxiety, which reduces stress hormones and the calorie-to-fat conversion. It was reported from a study that was done at Carnegie Mellon University that 25 minutes of meditation, which is done in three consecutive days, can remarkably reduce psychological stress (Creswell et al., 2014).

Stress could be one reason why dieting and exercising alone may not cause weight loss as expected. Most diets and exercise regimes enforce abrupt changes in people's ways of life, a state which can make them find it difficult to cope, thereby raising stress levels. Meditation helps individuals willingly accept healthy behaviors so that if they should, they diet and exercise with passion. At the end of the day, there are no stress hormones to counter their efforts to reduce weight.

Meditation is a form of training for both the mind and the body (Young, 2016). Significant improvement of attention, emotional regulation, creativity, and self-control is also attributed to meditation. People who engage in meditation can control their cravings than those that do not. Those who practice meditation find it easier to decide not to eat even when everyone else is. Meditation gives individuals better control of their lives.

Mindful Meditation as a Tool for Weight Loss

As presented by research studies, mindful meditation turns out to be the most effective when it comes to weight loss. In this section, I present some of the studies that support this notion.

Mindfulness-based interventions effectively reduce weight: In one study done by Carrière and colleagues (2017), a review of information that was reported by various studies on the efficacy of mindfulness-based interventions in reducing weight was done. Eighteen publications were used in this study. Analysis of the results from these publications confirmed that techniques based on mindfulness, such as mindful meditation, can cause significant weight loss. However, studies whose participants used both formal and informal meditation practices had greater effects on weight loss than those whose participants used formal meditation only. Apart from reducing weight, the review also revealed that mindfulness-based interventions alter eating behaviors related with obesity and overweight.

Meditation affects the physiological markers of stress: In another study (Pascoe, 2017), a meta-analysis review was conducted which investigated how meditation interventions such as focused attention, as compared to active controls, affected the biomarkers of stress. Specific attention was given to physiological biomarkers such as blood pressure, lipids, cortisol, heart rate, and cytokine expression. The results showed that meditation reduced cortisol levels, heart rate, blood pressure, triglycerides, C-reactive protein, and tumor necrosis factor-alpha. Since meditation reduced the physiological factors of stress, this implies that meditation reduces stress levels. As alluded to earlier, stress plays a role in weight gain. Therefore, the reduction in stress levels reduces weight gain, thereby promoting weight loss. Other studies reported that C-reactive protein plays a role in aiding increase in body weight (Mediano et al., 2013. Meditation, therefore, reduces weight gain by decreasing the secretion of C-reactive protein by the liver.

Mindfulness meditation reduces binge and emotional eating: A systematic review was done to analyze the effects of mindfulness meditation on binge eating, emotional eating, and ultimately, weight loss (Katterman, 2014). The review based its analysis on 14 studies that investigated how mindfulness meditation impacted weight loss and emotional and binge eating. The results that were compiled in the review suggested that emotional eating and binge eating behaviors are significantly reduced by mindfulness meditation.

Having had the evidence that mindfulness meditation is effective in trimming weight, it is equally important to know how this happens.

- **Shame and guilt are removed:** When you struggle with emotional eating, there is a tendency that you end up feeling guilty or shameful. Meditation reduces stress, which is often the trigger for overeating. Moreover, it helps you distinguish the cases when you eat in response to stress versus when you eat as a response to hunger. This further helps you to attain a calm and mindful approach to eating.
- **It's successful, even in the long run:** The effectiveness of mindfulness meditation is more visible in the long run. Without meditation techniques, dieting and exercising can trim off some pounds, but usually not for long. On the other hand, some studies have shown that mindful meditation aids weight loss and keeps the shedded weight away for longer (Carrière et al., 2017).
- **Stress and inflammation levels are lowered:** As we have discussed earlier, mindfulness meditation lowers stress levels by reducing cortisol levels in the body. It also reduces inflammation by reducing the secretion of C-reactive protein. Both stress and inflammation are associated with increased body weight.
- **It provides better control over cravings:** Most of our cravings are due to stress. We usually respond to stress by eating as a way to address it. Instead of using overeating as a coping mechanism for stressful conditions, mindfulness meditation teaches us to notice and observe our emotions

without judging them. By so doing, we refrain from overeating, which is a factor that promotes weight gain.

How to Start Meditating

After posting on social media that she had lost more than 30 pounds (13.6 kilograms) of weight without being conscious of it, Jennifer Marut was contacted by a countless number of ladies around the globe who needed to know how she did it. Jennifer testified that she could feel the desperation in their voices and deduce that they must have tried many other options to lose weight. She said, "I lost weight because I'd started meditating. That is the concrete foundation of it all. Many felt baffled by my answer, but it was because of my meditation practice that I naturally made lifestyle changes that led me to lose the extra weight I was not even aware I was carrying around" (Marut, 2019). Do you want to make your own success story out of Jennifer's? Let's explore more meditation practices that you can engage in.

Roll Breathing

Roll breathing is a belly breathing technique that is coupled with higher levels of self-awareness and breathing control. Regular practice alleviates stress and anxiety while also trimming down the weight. To do roll breathing, follow this procedure:

1. Sit or lie down on a mat, rug, or folded blanket.
2. Place your right hand on your chest and the left one on your belly.
3. Through your nose, deeply breathe into your belly and then breathe out through your mouth. Go through this cycle 10 times, ensuring that your chest does not move, but your belly can.

4. Breathe into your belly before you direct the air into your chest. Begin to release the air from the chest first, and then from your belly. Stick to this pattern of breathing for five minutes (Lawrence, 2020).

Deep Breathing

Deep breathing promotes weight loss by boosting your metabolism. It ensures that oxygen is available to body cells for use in body processes and removes toxic wastes from the body. Let's do some deep breathing meditation.

1. Sit on a mat in a position that keeps your spinal cord straight. Place your hands on your knees to keep them relaxed.
2. Breathe into your belly using your nose. Count to five while you do this. Can you feel your belly filled with air?
3. Hold your breath for two counts before you begin to breathe out as you count to five. Can you feel the emptiness in your belly?
4. Repeat steps one to three about 10 times.

Chakra Meditation

Chakra is a Sanskrit word, which means "wheel" or "disk." In meditation, these wheels or disks are for spinning energy in energy centers within the human body. Each energy center corresponds to a specific group of nerves or body organs. Therefore, chakra meditation activates the energy points situated along with your head and spine, including the throat, crown, heart, root, sacral, solar plexus, and third-eye. It is reported that solar plexus meditation is associated with weight loss (Lawrence, 2020). The solar plexus is in your upper abdomen.

To do solar plexus chakra meditation, follow these steps:

1. Sit down on a mat. Place your hands on your thighs with the palms facing upwards, and close your eyes.
2. Imagine a warm and bright yellow light, gradually filling your whole body. The solar plexus is yellow, which is the reason why you should visualize a yellow light.
3. Once the light reaches your upper abdomen, stop it and hold it there. Notice the relaxing feeling that is brought by this new energy.
4. As you continue to visualize, see the yellow light spilling onto the ground, after which it returns to your body again. Imagine this as many times as you can.
5. End the meditation session by letting the yellow light fall to the ground, and then open your eyes.

Morning Breathing Meditation

This meditation technique is a good way to begin a new day as it clears any clogged air passages. It also relaxes stiffened muscles. Here is how to do morning breathing meditation:

1. While standing, let your upper body fall forward. Your knees should be slightly bent, and your hands should fall in a relaxed manner by your sides.
2. Take a deep breath through your nose and simultaneously roll up gradually until you stand up again.
3. While still standing, hold your breath for six seconds.
4. Begin to breathe out while you simultaneously bend over to the position that you were in step 1.
5. Repeat steps one to four at least seven times.

Guided Imagery

If you do not prefer breathing exercises, guided imagery is a great alternative. Guided imagery involves the visualization of a dream place and uses that to derive peace within you. Besides relieving pain and tension, guided imagery can contribute to weight loss.

Follow these steps for guided imagery meditation:

1. Sit down with your eyes closed.
2. Visualize a beautiful and peaceful place and see yourself in that place.
3. Using your five senses, begin to add some detail to the view that you are seeing. For example, *hear* some singing birds, *feel* the peaceful breeze, *pluck* some flowers, and *smell* their fragrance.
4. To conclude, take two deep breaths and open your eyes.

4-7-8 Breathing

This is another form of belly breathing, which is good for enhancing a calm and relaxed state. Follow the procedure described below and enjoy the experience of 4-7-8 breathing meditation.

1. You can either sit or lie down in whichever position is comfortable for you.
2. Use the tip of your tongue to touch your upper teeth.
3. While you count up to four, breath in through your nose.
4. Hold your breath for seven counts.
5. Without changing the position of your tongue, breathe out through your mouth while you count up to 8.
6. Repeat steps one to five at least seven times.

Yoga Meditation

Unlike the other meditation techniques that we described before, yoga meditation does not require you to sit or lie still. Rather, you should adopt a yoga pose that you maintain while you meditate. Yoga meditation reduces weight, anxiety, and chronic pain. It also promotes mindful eating, which in turn reduces bad eating habits such as binge eating. You can build muscle using yoga meditation, which also contributes to weight loss (Lawrence, 2020). Let's explore the different poses that you can consider for yoga meditation.

Upward-facing dog: Lie down on your belly. Press your arms to the floor so that your fingers are facing forward. Begin to lift your upper body up, until your hands are straight. Concentrate on your breathing while you are in this position, making sure that your navel does not touch the floor.

Tree pose: Take a standing position and shift your weight slightly to your left leg. Bend your right leg inward, grab it by the ankle, and place it on the inner thigh of your left leg so that your left leg's inner thigh will be in contact with the sole of your right leg's foot. Keep your upper body upright and maintain your balance. Now, place your arms together in a "prayer pose," close your eyes, and begin to breathe in and out slowly. You can also try guided imagery or breathing exercises in this pose.

Triangle pose: Turn your right foot inward and your left foot to the left. Breathe in while you raise your hands so that they extend to your sides. While you exhale, let your left arm get down and touch your left foot's toes, or at least, your ankle. That means your body would have bent towards the left for you to be able to do this. Now, raise your right leg towards the ceiling as much as you can. Each time you breathe in, lift your torso, and twist your body when you breathe out so that you stay mindful.

Chapter 5:

Practicing Motivation: How Not to

Give Up

How many times have you tried to lose weight, yet, all efforts ended up in vain? Was it once, thrice, ten times or you have lost count? At one time, you embarked on weight loss endeavors probably because you were tired of being identified as "that fat lady." Maybe it was because you were getting ready for the get-together party with your high school friends, and you wanted them to see you as that slim and hot chick that you were during the "heydays." Alternatively, you admired a friend's new shape after successful efforts to lose weight. After a few weeks of maintaining the zeal to exercise and watch your diet, you noticed that you had shed a few pounds. This probably raised your hopes and made you feel like you were getting there. You don't quite remember what happened after that. All that you remember was the frustrating "scale day" when you realized that you had gained more pounds, even more than the ones you lost in the first place.

The truth of the matter is that you lost your motivation somewhere along the way, and you slipped back to your old, unhealthy lifestyle. In other words, your motivation was short-lived, either because it was not strong enough or was rooted in short-lived goals. A good example of a short-lived motivation is the scenario that we gave above, where one targets losing weight for, say, a particular event. Once the event is over, the reason for losing weight also disappears. Therefore, motivation is a factor of paramount importance as far as the journey to losing weight is concerned. This chapter explores activities and techniques that can help individuals increase and maintain their motivation before and after achieving their targets for losing weight.

Categories of Weight Loss Motivation

There are two categories of motivation that can be used when one intends to lose weight. These are intrinsic and extrinsic motivation (Livingstone, 2019), and we will explore these further in this section.

Extrinsic Motivation

Extrinsic motivation is derived from outside oneself and is, therefore, external. This type of motivation is usually focused on rewards or avoidance of unwanted results. Therefore, you engage in a certain behavior not because you enjoy the process, but because of what you will get if you do it. For example, when the sole reason for altering your eating patterns and food choice is to lose weight, then the motivation is extrinsic. Most drastic weight loss plans such as extreme diet changes and fasting are part of extrinsic motivation.

Extrinsic motivation provides a great push to start making efforts to lose weight and can even bring quick results in the best-case scenario. However, this type of motivation quickly dies off when there is a change in motivation or when, for some reason, the motivation becomes absent. In other words, extrinsic motivation is more effective in short-term weight loss goals but cannot be fully-trusted with long-term goals of losing weight. Some research suggests that extrinsically motivated people always switch between external motives, even if they continue to fail them. At the end of the day, they swing between losing weight a little bit and regaining it.

Extrinsic motivation is further categorized into guilt avoidance and people-pleasing. *People-pleasing motivation* is based on the longing to gain approval from others. It usually takes its stand when you start making efforts to lose weight based on the fact that someone else, be it a parent, friend, relative, or colleague, showed that they dislike or disapprove of your body. Again, when the motive is to make sure that someone should say, "My goodness, is this you!" then it is extrinsic.

The danger of this type of motivation is that when you finally lose the weight and don't get much of that "Wow!" experience you were expecting, you are more likely to lose the zeal and return to binging, emotional eating, and other unhealthy activities. Before you know it, you will be back to point zero.

Guilt avoidance becomes the motive when you want to lose weight because you want to be like everyone else and fit in the groups within society without the feeling that something is wrong with you. To simply put it, you will feel like there is a certain way you should look according to society. Therefore, to look like what is expected, you would do anything to help you achieve it.

Intrinsic Motivation

Intrinsic motivation emanates from within an individual, which is why it is also called internal motivation. It is based on meaningful reasons for losing weight, which acknowledges that the journey will not be necessarily easy, but still cultivates inner interest and enjoyment in losing weight. Intrinsic motivation does not only create joy upon achieving your target weight but makes the journey towards the achievement an enjoyable accomplishment on its own.

Since it emanates from within you, intrinsic motivation is reliable in achieving long term goals of losing weight, let alone maintaining them. The consistency that intrinsic motivation brings is that people who are motivated from within tend to be concerned about maintaining a healthy lifestyle more. They then reap the benefits such as weight loss in the process. It is also easier for such people to maintain their desired weight because reaching their target weight does not make them give up the healthy lifestyle that they would have attained. They celebrate the weight loss achievement, not as a destination, but as a benefit of living a healthy lifestyle, motivating them to continue.

Three feelings help individuals create intrinsic motivation within themselves so that they attain a change of behavior that carries them beyond achieving their weight-loss goal:

- **Autonomy:** One should feel like they decided to embark on the journey to lose weight on their own, without coercion from extrinsic factors. If they should choose any dietary routines, their motivation to stick to them is derived from within.
- **Competence:** One must feel confident that they will go through the required changes in their day-to-day lifestyle and achieve their goal of losing weight in the process.
- **Relatedness:** Usually, some people support you in your weight loss goals. The feeling of belonging and acceptance with such people cultivates intrinsic motivation. Support is only reliable and unharmful if it does not require accountability, dependency, and sponsorship (Livingstone, 2019). You should not feel obliged to report to anyone about your progress; neither should you depend on someone to sponsor you to achieve the goal. However, communities that support a person's individual goals and help them get back up if they fall along the way are of paramount importance. Relatedness supports the concept of interdependence, which acknowledges that even though we can possibly do without each other, we can accomplish more and even better when we work together (Covey & Covey, 2020).

Important Considerations

Having understood the types of weight loss motivation that are associated with weight loss, it is also important to consider the following ideas as they will guide you into creating the right motivation that will take you through your weight loss journey:

- You should be completely sure that the dietary style you choose is manageable, even in the long run. If not, it may end up being another stressor, which will cause you to gain more weight instead of losing weight. Moreover, the dietary style of your choice should be able to bring the desired results.

- Everything about the dietary style or exercise regime that you embark on should be utterly your own choice, without coercion or being imposed on you by anyone. This includes the starting date and goal.
- Look for a community of supporters that will boost your morale without overlapping with your autonomy.

How to Create Motivation in Yourself

Weight loss is not something that you can achieve effortlessly. It calls for your patience, focus, persistence, self-control, and motivation. Your success in losing weight is highly dependent on the extent to which you remain motivated along the way. You need the motivation that will take you all the way to your goal and even beyond so that you will be able to maintain your desired weight. Motivation can be created, recreated if lost or even improved. This section focuses on techniques that boost your motivation.

Believe in Yourself

The abundance of diets and exercise regimes that people are using to lose weight is, to some extent, leading to demotivation in some people. The demotivation arises from the fact that most diets end up failing to promote long-term loss of weight. After trying and failing many times, many people find it difficult to believe that they can still lose weight. Therefore, even when they embark on other endeavors that may possibly work, they try them, but with some reservations. Losing weight is a goal that you can achieve when you believe in yourself and tell yourself that you can do it. You will need to learn to take charge of what you eat, as well as your eating habits, for you to increase your self-confidence.

Be Clear on Your Reasons

The reasons why you decided to lose weight can be your great motivation if you set them right and honestly. Identify the reasons why you chose to lose weight and explain why they are. You can even write down a list and always remind yourself of these reasons. Your reasons could be, "I need to lose 55 pounds within the next 18 months so that I will look good on my graduation." Keep the list handy by having a copy in your wallet, smartphone, or anywhere else where you can easily access it when you need motivation. Good reasons can be a good motivation when your old unhealthy lifestyles begin to reappear.

Your Goals and Expectation Should be Realistic

One of the things that kill motivation is unrealistic and unreasonable goals. Dawn Jackson Blatner, author of the Flexitarian diet, once said, "I see so many women in my private practice for weight loss, and no matter their age, most have unreasonable weight loss goals" (CFS Fitness Staff, n.d). Trying to lose 20 pounds per week in normal everyday life is an unrealistic goal. Normally, an average person burns up to 2,200 calories in one day. On the other hand, you must burn 3,500 calories more than you eat if you must lose a pound of weight. Therefore, you will have to consume 1,000 fewer calories than you burn per day for you to lose two pounds in a week (CFS Fitness Staff, n.d). Now, imagine if the goal to lose 20 pounds in a week is feasible. That is a concern because the stress that is posed by trying to achieve goals that are, in fact, not achievable counters the weight-loss efforts. Plan your goals well, and put realistic, achievable, and measurable goals in place.

Refrain From Criticizing Yourself

Even after setting realistic goals, mistakes and failures are often inevitable. However, the solution is not punishing yourself and telling yourself that you are not good enough. Besides thwarting your self-confidence, criticizing yourself raises stress and anxiety levels, both of which are factors that aid weight gain through the action of hormones such as cortisol and adrenaline. These hormones slow down metabolism and promote the conversion of calories to fats. Some cravings for unhealthy foods are a response to stress. Therefore, instead of losing weight, you might gain it if you allow self-criticism to have a place. Give yourself positive assurances that you are well able to reach your goal, no matter the challenges and failures along the way.

Begin Each Day With a Motivational Phrase

One study tested various motivational practices on 44,000 participants, and the study revealed that self-affirmation had the best results (Best Life Editors, 2017). Therefore, telling yourself some self-motivating statements every morning is a great way to begin your day. You could tell yourself, "This is another chance for me to conquer," or "I choose to be positive in everything that I will do today." Such statements will motivate you to remain focused on achieving your goals, including losing weight.

It's Not All About Losing Weight

This sounds a bit confusing, right? No need to worry; I will clarify it for you. Quite often, we focus on seeing lower numbers when we get onto the scale. That is when we get satisfied that we are getting healthier. However, the main focus should rather be on losing fat, which can sometimes happen without significantly impacting the number of pounds. I will explain this with an example. Suppose you lose 25 pounds of calories and gain 20 pounds of muscle. You can easily get frustrated when you get onto the scale because the scale will show you that you lost 5 pounds when the other 20 pounds were countered by the growth in muscle.

When you workout to burn calories, which your body cannot get from food intake, the body turns to fat reserves and the muscles. As a result, you will lose fat while your muscle becomes leaner and denser, with no superfluous fat. This helps your muscles become stronger so that you can exercise better and burn even more calories. This is an ideal situation. Instead of depending on counting pounds, check yourself in the mirror; it will tell a better story. More ideally, you can measure around your arms, neck, belly, hips, abdomen, and thighs so that you can compare them after every week. With this, you will notice that you are making progress.

Derive Honest Appreciation for Your Body

When was the last time you looked at yourself in the mirror? Not looking in the mirror is not a way to escape the fact that you are probably overweight. It only makes you overlook that fact, and you end up continually neglecting your well-being through unhealthy lifestyles. Look at the mirror. The lady you see needs to be appreciated by you. Tell yourself something good, not to pamper and deceive yourself, but honestly. The size of your body is not everything about you. The moment that you learn to appreciate the good things about yourself, you will show yourself more love by taking care of yourself through healthier eating and living.

Steer Clear of "Clever Tricks" and Diet Fads

The internet is currently clogged with diets with tricks and gimmicks embedded in them to convince desperate people to try them for dramatic weight loss. The truth of the matter is that usually, they do not work. Such diets are called fad diets, and they are sometimes based on drinking a certain juice or leaving out a certain food in your diet. Diet fads are not only detrimental to your health; they do not guarantee long-term weight loss. It may not work at all, or if it does, the weight loss is short-lived. The failures and disappointments associated with diet fads thwart your motivation, and the more failures you encounter, the more difficult it becomes to keep back up. Adopt a steady and healthy lifestyle that will reduce your weight gradually and realistically. This keeps your body healthy and maintains your weight loss efforts even in the long run.

Include More Fibre in Your Diet

Lentils, chickpeas, and steel-cut oats are fiber-rich foods that you can consider including in your diet. Fiber is effective in aiding weight loss. Besides keeping your gut microorganisms healthy, fibers also reduce your appetite by keeping you fuller for longer. This reduces your daily food consumption.

Create and Maintain Supportive Relationships

Being part of a group that has the same goal of losing weight the healthy way can be extremely motivating. This could be with friends, colleagues, or an association in the neighborhood. Your family can be the best cheerleaders if you prove serious and show that you are bent on losing weight. If you cannot get face-to-face support in your neighborhood, remote support is another viable option. Some studies have shown that people who receive support over the phone showed similar results to those who received in-person support (CFS Fitness Staff, 2020). Moreover, every support group that you may choose to join was created by someone, so you can also create your own support group and let others with the same goal as yours join you.

Eat a Protein-Rich Breakfast

A breakfast that is rich in protein, especially whey protein, is a great start for a new day and a sustainable motivation in your endeavors to lose weight. A protein-rich breakfast makes you feel fuller for the rest of the day. As a result, by the time you sleep, you would have eaten less. Besides, it provides you with more energy for all your activities, and you won't feel drained should you decide to work out.

Refrain From Fashion and Fitness Magazines

When you read fashion and fitness magazines and see good looking fitness models, an emotional response is triggered in you, which feels like motivation. This kind of motivation is brief because it has nothing to do with how those models obtained the body shape that you see. The motivation is not only external but also what I would like to call "surface" motivation, which can easily disappear. If you should use someone as a motivation for your goal, then it should be someone who has gone through and overcame difficulties and obstacles, which you are aware of. Such motivation is long-term and can keep you going when you feel discouraged.

Make Short-Term Goals

Theodora Blanchfiels, the author of *Preppy Runner*, said, "So you can't run a mile now? That's okay. Start out walking. You'll get to running, I promise. Take things one step at a time. I started out with 15 minutes of intervals on the treadmill in February. Next weekend, I am running a half-marathon" (CFS Fitness Staff, 2020). While you would want to achieve the long term goal of losing weight and maintaining it, you might find it easier to accomplish that if you set objectives or short-term goals that will collectively make your ultimate goal a reality. Focusing on your two-year goal is more difficult than concentrating on, say, one-week goals that contribute to your long-term goal. It saves you the exhaustion that comes with the long journey of losing weight.

Slow Down Your Eating

One research revealed that people who ate their food faster hadn't higher body mass index than those that ate at a slower pace (Best Life Editors, 2017). When you eat slowly, it is easier to realize when you are full, while you tend to enjoy the food better since it is easier to involve all your senses. When you eat quicker, you are more likely to overeat.

The tendency to rush when you are eating is sometimes due to not eating your meals on time. Suppose you eat your breakfast late, and you have to go to work, or you eat your lunch late, while you have to be in a meeting by the end of the lunch hour. You see the picture, right? To avoid such scenarios, eat your meals on time. Another study showed that people who eat their lunch within the lunch hour lose more weight than those who miss the lunch hour and eat their lunch later in the day (Best Life Editors, 2017). Therefore, by eating your meals on time, you kill two birds with one stone because you will also be able to eat at a slower pace.

Embrace What You Are Striving For

Could it be that you want to lose weight so that you can stick around longer and have more time with your family, or even see your grandchildren? Could it be because you want to fit in your favorite dress that you wore on your graduation day years back? Whatever the reason could be, do not wait until you lose weight before you start spending quality time with your family. Do not hide the dress with the shame that you can't fit into it; place it where you can see it to motivate you towards the day when you will wear it. Keep embracing what losing weight will help you to achieve.

Give Room for Setbacks

While the ultimate goal is not to fail, small failures along your weight loss journey are inevitable. Expecting success all the way can lead to frustration or even ultimate failure as individuals find it difficult to accept disappointments. Planning and accepting failures is a step toward conquering them. Be realistic to the fact that you are not "superman." There are times when you can't focus on the goal, and that's normal. When you plan to begin your weight loss journey, don't expect perfection, but include the inevitable small failures so that they do not take you by surprise, neither should they take you down. Denis Waitley said, "Failure should be our teacher, not our undertaker. Failure is a delay, not defeat. It is a temporary detour, not a dead end. Failure is something we can avoid only by saying nothing, doing nothing, and being nothing" (Walter, n.d.). As long as you are doing something meaningful, intermittent failure is inevitable.

Allow Yourself to Eat the Food That You Enjoy

Most diets are restrictive, and they stop you from eating even the foods that you enjoy eating. Weight loss is not all about completely refraining from eating the foods that you enjoy, even those that we often label as bad, unhealthy, or banned. It all depends on how much you eat and the frequency at which you eat the food. Completely refraining from the food you enjoy will only increase your cravings for it so that you end up eating more than you could have eaten if you had not restricted yourself. Therefore, once in a while, you should give in to your cravings. This makes any other efforts that you make to lose weight more of a pleasure than a chore. A successful weight loss journey is possible when you adopt a sustainable and non stressful way of eating that you will naturally enjoy. Restricting yourself to some diets may not be enjoyable, especially in the long run.

Acquire Knowledge About Nutrition

"Do not eat fats; they are bad for your health." You have probably come across similar statements a couple of times. This is a wave of information that has filled the internet and other dietary media and has created "fatphobia" in many people. Fats are an important part of our diet, and completely refraining from eating them is equally unhealthy. In fact, dietary fat keeps us feeling fuller for longer. This reduces our appetite for food than how carbohydrates and low-fat foods would. It is, however, important that you monitor the amounts of fats that you take. Knowledge of such dietary information helps you select food based on the understanding of what happens at the physiological level, rather than just making decisions based on what is stipulated in diets.

Better Your Relationship With Food

How is your relationship with food? Do you take charge of the food you eat, or does it control you? There are many factors that determine your relationship with food, and these include:

- Whether you conceive yourself with love or criticism
- Your history of growing up and upbringing
- The extent to which you rely on food to cope with stressful situations
- Whether you have mental health problems such as depression and anxiety
- The things that trigger you to make poor food choices
- Whether you live a stressful life or not
- Whether you are emotionally stable or can easily burst emotionally
- Your personality, whether you are a perfectionist, good planner, people-pleaser, flexible, or rigid

No matter the factors that affect the way you relate to food, you can choose to take charge by learning to practice mindful eating. A better relationship with food is a great motivation to lose weight.

Take Care of Yourself

Even when you control your eating habits, other factors of your lifestyle, such as high-stress levels and poor sleeping habits, can have counter-effects on losing weight. Identify the stressors in your life so that you can address them accordingly. You equally need enough time to rest so that you keep your mind alert. When you take good care of yourself, you tend to make better choices on food consumption. You are also better able to sustain your motivation towards achieving goals.

Don't Let Your Life Be All About Weight Loss

While losing weight is an important aspect of your life, it is not all that matters. Do not let your life revolve around losing weight and nothing else. The weight loss journey will become hectic if you do that. Give yourself a break from focusing on weight loss, and occupy yourself with other things such as helping a neighbor paint their house, cleaning your house, or learning some new skills. This could be sewing, embroidery, making home-made shampoo, and even playing "hide and seek" with your children. Build and maintain relationships, have fun and laugh, without allowing the term "weight loss" to peep through your mind.

Chapter 6:

Losing Weight With Positive

Thoughts

Susan, a young lady in her twenties, had always used positive thoughts in all her endeavors, and they came to pass, just the way she liked it. She never imagined herself using this art of thinking positively about herself as a tool for losing weight, at least not until she noticed that she had gained weight more than she had ever done on her biggest "self." Reaching 170 pounds from her ideal weight of 139 pounds got her worried and focused on shedding the extra weight. She decided to speak to herself that she would lose weight, specifically a pound a day.

The amazing part is that Susan told herself that she would lose this weight while eating whatever she wanted. Sounds impossible, doesn't it? She would say to herself while eating her food, "The food that I eat nourishes my body and keeps me thin and in my perfect form." Here and there, she would feel a little bit guilty for eating a piece of chocolate, and she would then tell herself that she needed to eat something healthy because she would have *eaten a piece of chocolate in the morning*, to make herself forget that it ever happened. The best part of the story is that she did lose a pound each day! (Susan, n.d.).

There is a close association between what we think about ourselves and what happens in our lives. When you look at yourself in the mirror, what you think about yourself determines whether you will lose or gain weight. You gain weight when you think negatively about yourself, even when you pretend to say good things contrary to what you think. Your thoughts and beliefs are what matters. Weight gain comes as a result of one negative thought that gave birth to more negative thoughts. In the same manner, just a single positive thought is all you need to start losing weight.

Supporting Scientific Evidence

There is scientific evidence, which supports the fact that the mindset plays a crucial role in losing weight. In a study done by Crum and Langer (2007), an analysis of whether the mindset has a role to play in the relationship between exercise and health was done. The participants in the study were 84 hotel attendants who were separated into informed and uninformed groups. The informed group was told that their work was good enough exercise, and they, therefore, led active lives. They were also provided with examples of how the day-to-day responsibilities of their work were a form of exercise. Nothing was told to the "uniformed" group. At the end of four weeks of the study, a significant decrease in weight, body mass index, blood pressure, waist-to-hip ratio, and body fat were observed in participants that were in the "informed" group compared to the "uniformed" participants. The reason for this difference was that the "informed" participants of the study believed that they were doing a lot of exercise even though there was no change in their actual physical activity. It was concluded from this study that the mindset plays a role in how exercise affects health.

In the study that has been described above, the information that was given to the participants that were in the "informed" group changed their mindsets towards their jobs. Whenever they were doing their work, they were positive that they were exercising. Therefore, even though they did not change the way they were doing their work, the body decided that they were exercising because of what they were thinking, and so, they lost weight. Those who had not been given any information about their work being some form of exercise had no change in mindset; therefore, not much change was realized in the physiological markers for weight loss. If your goal is to lose weight, what you think determines whether you will succeed.

The Law of Attraction

Positive thinking is highly based on the Law of Attraction. The Law of Attraction is a manifestation force that attracts and brings into our lives, anything that we focus our thoughts and beliefs on (Power of Positivity, 2018). It is a principle that emphasizes that you attract what you are, in terms of thoughts, actions, beliefs, and feelings. The Law of Attraction states that "like attracts like." When all the factors that define you are put together, they determine the frequency at which you energetically vibrate. The people, achievements, circumstances, situations, and other things that become associated with your life are those that align to the frequency at which you vibrate. If you are resentful and forgiving, whatever that is attracted to your life is associated with resentment and unforgiveness, even the people. When love becomes your focal point, you also attract loving people, situations, and circumstances. You attract things that match your being, be it positively or negatively.

The events and circumstances that we encounter in our lives always have various meanings and interpretations. If one situation is presented to different people, they are all more likely to interpret the same situation differently, depending on their perceptions, experiences, thoughts, and beliefs. The interpretations that an individual may have concerning a situation determine how they will react to that situation. Therefore, to induce the reaction that you prefer for a particular situation, check how you interpret it. Positive interpretations yield positive reactions. To interpret situations positively, you should alter your thoughts, beliefs, attitudes, and feelings towards positivity.

Love and gratitude for yourself and your body are powerful factors that attract weight loss (Daniels, 2013). They can undo any thoughts of resentment, regret, hatred, and unappreciation that you have for your body, which may have already manifested as weight gain. Shower yourself with excess love and appreciation for who you are, and you will notice inches falling off your waist and pounds dropping overall. See yourself as the person you have always wanted to be, and positivity will progressively develop in you.

According to the Law of Attraction, the body responds to your genuine thoughts. This means that if you say, "I am so grateful for who I am," when your thoughts are saying the opposite, your body will respond to your thoughts instead. Therefore, you should train your mind to think positively about your goal of losing weight. Consider the following as you use the Law of Attraction to lose weight:

- Visualize yourself as having lost weight already and maintain that vibration frequency by living as though you have reached your weight target. This grows the love and appreciation for the body you want by believing that you already have it.
- Reinforce your belief by loudly speaking out positive words of gratitude like, "I am grateful for my slender, healthy, and strong body."
- Focus on the good things that you have in your life to cultivate the spirit of gratitude in you.
- Surround yourself with "heart" energy. I will explain more about heart energy in the next section.

Mind and Heart Energy

All your experiences in life are created by positive and negative thoughts through the Law of Attraction. The words that you speak are, therefore, a result of your thoughts. In other words, the power to create that is embedded in your words is derived from your thoughts. Therefore, by controlling your thoughts, you control your life. This controlled energy that is derived from your mind is called *mind energy*. Controlling your thoughts, removing limiting beliefs, and reprogramming your subconscious mind requires mind energy (Daniel, 2012). Using mind energy requires your own effort, should it work.

If you need to achieve your weight loss goals more effortlessly, the Law of Attraction introduces another form of energy called *heart energy*, which is also referred to as the energy of the Universe. According to Daniel (2020), heart energy is the secret of the Law of Attraction, which can help you lose weight even more. Heart energy provides your thoughts with the energy to come to life. The most powerful and effective type of heart energy is love. For heart energy to work in your weight-loss goals, you should focus on the following:

- Let love be associated with every thought that you have concerning your goal to lose weight. You should love the idea, the process, and the result of losing weight.
- Visualize and feel the love surrounding you. This way, you will appreciate yourself more.
- Feel love for everyone and everything, and take them as allies to achieving your goals.

You cannot master these things in a single day; you will need continual practice. With time, you will notice that they will begin to come out more naturally, with less effort.

Manifesting Your Reality Through the Law of Attraction

Knowing about the Law of Attraction is not enough. You need to learn how to use this law to make your weight-loss goals come to reality. This section provides you with practical ways to apply the Law of Attraction as a tool for losing weight.

Clarify the Reasons Why You Want to Lose Weight

All the success stories of people who used the Law of Attraction to lose weight have one thing in common; they had clear answers to this question: Why do you want to lose weight? These reasons are your aims, and they usually align with your beliefs. According to the Law of Attraction, if your reasons and beliefs are negative, losing weight will be difficult. Negative reasons are often associated with emotions such as resentment, hatred, insecurity, and lack (Hurst, n.d.). If you choose to lose weight because your husband left you for a slender lady, then the reasons are based on competition and emotions such as jealousy, resentment, and possibly hatred. Such emotions cause you to vibrate at a frequency that attracts negative things, which are opposite to what you want. You are even more likely to gain weight.

Your reasons for losing weight should be created from a view-point of self-respect, growth, development, and positivity. For example, you can choose to lose weight because you want to avoid diseases associated with excess weight, such as stroke, coronary heart disease, hypertension, and type 2 diabetes. Positive reasons like these are associated with positive feelings that promote the manifestation of weight loss.

Be Attentive to Your Thoughts

Pain, frustration, feelings of unacceptance, grief, and lack are circumstances that are inevitable. This is why stress is always part of our lives. While there are some stressors that we can avoid, most of them are natural and unavoidable. However, we can choose how we react to stress so that it does not determine our behavior. We can only positively react to stress when we can control what we think, which is equally an uneasy task. When you can ensure that stress doesn't control your thoughts, you equally control it from influencing your behavior, which is the best thing you can do to lose weight. Most emotional eating is in response to stressful conditions, and it leads to overeating, which in turn promotes weight gain. The more you can control behaviors associated with stress, such as emotional eating, the more control you have over your weight.

You might be asking, "How do I stop stress from influencing my thoughts and behavior?" There are many methods through which you can control the way stress influences your thoughts and behavior. These include:

- **Journaling:** This involves writing down what you think and feel on a piece of paper, book, or on your smartphone so that you can analyze and understand yourself better. Writing your thoughts and feelings exposes them, and this helps you find ways to control them.
- **Meditation:** Through meditation, you achieve a deep state of relaxation that calms any thoughts associated with stress. It trains your mind to focus on the present moment, thereby alleviating stressful thoughts associated with your past and future.
- **Prayer:** In this case, individuals stop focusing on stressors and their effects but submit them to God using the doctrines that they believe in, through prayer, trusting that their stressful situations will be solved. That way, they feel relieved through the belief that whatever was causing their stress and the stress itself would have been taken off their lives.
- **Yoga:** Some of the ways through which yoga controls stress are lifting your mood and increasing mindfulness and self-compassion. It also increases a sense of emotional and physical well-being. One study showed that people who practice yoga have better tolerance to pain because their bodies can regulate responses to stress (Harvard Health Publishing, 2018).
- **Talking to someone:** In most cases, we tend to think amiss and negatively when we are stressed. Talking to someone familiar with your situation through their own personal experiences can be of great help in maintaining positivity. In this case, you may stop thinking positively or negatively and use

the "borrowed positivity" from the person that you choose to talk to until you feel better.

- **Positive thinking:** This is done by changing the way you perceive the stress that is affecting you. A study carried out by Allia Cram and colleagues on how mindsets affect the way our bodies respond to stress. The results from the study brought the researchers to the conclusion that an individual's mindset towards stress determines the body's response to it (Cram et al., 2013). Unfortunately, most sources of information reinforce the concept that stress is always bad, which is not necessarily true. Stress can boost your memory and help you accomplish tasks more efficiently. It is also a crucial warning system, which produces the fight-or-flight response. When we perceive stress as good for us, our bodies respond in a way that helps us overcome the stress (Kabir, n.d.).

Naturally, our minds want to focus on negative things, no wonder why negative things seem to be shouty compared to positive ones. For example, if you have been successfully eating healthily and leading an active life for, say, six months, a single day of binging may make your mind paint the whole journey that you travelled for the past six months as a failure. We naturally recognize the negative things more. That is why being positive requires much effort to shift the mind from what it is used to, that is, thinking negatively. Thinking positively sometimes requires you not to focus on the stimuli from the environment. It involves speaking against what you see coming.

Love Your Body

Simple logic would assume that there is no point in claiming that you love the body you are making all efforts to change. Well, if you want to lose weight using positive thinking, you should love your current body. By the way, it's not like there is nothing good about your current body; it's just that you want to lose weight. Identify the good things about your body and be grateful for what you are and what you can accomplish right now. Show yourself some self-love by:

- Creating a list of at least 10 things your body can do now, even the simplest skills you usually took for granted. If there are bigger things, include them in the list because they provide even greater motivation.
- Be your own guest and treat yourself with love. Feed yourself healthily, give yourself enough time to rest and sleep, keep your body clean, or give your body a massage in appreciation.
- Refrain from comparing yourself with anyone else because, if you do, you become prone to criticizing your body and give room for negative emotions such as envy. Always remind yourself that you are unique in your own way, and no one can take your place.
- Dress your body the way you want it to look when you finally lose weight. There is no need for you to wait until you have reached your target weight before you can show yourself that love.

Self-Awareness Is Key

Rather than simply focusing on weight loss, take time to consider other factors that come with your efforts to lose weight. For instance, you could consider yourself more active than people who are not worried about losing weight. Studies report that people who believe they are active tend to lose weight faster, even when there is no actual increase in their physical activity (Crum & Langer, 2007). The positivity that is associated with thinking that you are doing something that enhances your health is what aids the desired weight loss. Think, see and talk of yourself as an energetic and active lady who is losing weight, and that is what you will attract into your life.

Weight Loss Does Not Define the Whole of Your Health Journey

 We often define our health based on weight loss, making weight loss the destination in our health journey. This is a misconception. It is important to note that your health journey never ends as long as you are still alive. You should regard weight loss as part of your health journey if you want to manifest weight loss through the Law of Attraction.

Like any other journey, it is unlikely that your weight-loss journey will be straight and smooth. You may fail to keep up with what you originally planned concerning your eating routines, here and there, or even completely. It is all part of the journey, but keep it at the back of your mind that you can achieve whatever you set your mind to do. Moreover, that does not mean that you have failed the obligation to keep yourself healthy. Judging yourself only accommodates negative thoughts that manifest themselves as failures.

Factors such as fear do not only affect weight loss but your whole health journey. Fear can control you into eating what you wouldn't eat under normal circumstances. You could find yourself drinking alcohol because you are afraid, and you are trying to cope. Besides, fear is a negative vibe, which attracts negative things from the Universe. This affects your weight control endeavors. You cannot control your fears using things from outside forces like alcohol and food. The only way through which you can control your health is by controlling "you," not what is outside you.

Weight Loss Is a Symptom of Something Bigger

Do you really think that the reason why you are carrying some pounds you consider as "excess" is because you ate too much fat or carbohydrate? There is another underlying cause that led you into overeating, binge eating, and stress eating. Your excess weight is highly associated with the type of feelings that you accommodated all along, negative feelings to be precise. In other words, your weight represents what you have been feeling. Weight gain represents negative feelings, while weight loss is highly associated with positive feelings, as far as the law of attraction is concerned. Basically, weight gain reflects negative emotions, such as fear (Ball, 2020).

Change Your Relationship With Food

Give priority to the importance of food just as you prioritize the relationship with your body in your endeavors to lose weight. Take note of how you feel when you eat food. Are there any differences in the way you feel when you eat certain types of food? Do you feel guilty when you eat some food? If you often find yourself binge eating or emotional eating, you need to identify the causes, whether it is stress, anxiety, or anything else. Only when you can identify the causes of your unhealthy eating behaviors, will you make the relevant changes that help you stop them. It is important that you learn to dissociate food with negative emotions and align them with positivity. You can do this by paying special attention to how you prepare your food. For example, taking the time to prepare a fresh meal for yourself will cultivate better feelings towards the food than eating a microwaved meal (Hurst, n.d.).

Change Your Emotional State

Is it possible for you to feel both fear and gratitude? Certainly not. The moment you begin to appreciate yourself, fear disappears, and you send a positive vibe to the Universe. To successfully use the Law of Attraction to aid weight loss, you need to change the state of your emotions so that they align with positivity towards your weight-loss goal. Once you succeed in creating the right emotional state, the next thing would be to maintain it. That is what helps you maintain your desired weight when you reach your targeted weight. Charles Swindoll said, "Life is 10% of what happens to you and 90% of how you react to it" (Turaga, 2019). If you can direct your attitude to exhibit high levels of positivity, you can lose weight using the Law of Attraction, and succeed in other areas of your life as well.

Believe and trust God for the things that you cannot handle on your own. There is no way you can disregard shun emotions such as fear, frustration, boredom, anxiety, sadness, hate, and anger completely because they are natural emotions that come along with the gift of life. However, you can choose how you react to these emotions, so you don't give them the leeway to distort your positivity. Interestingly, the Law of Attraction and manifestation work, whether you are aware of it or not. What you have experienced so far in your endeavors to lose weight are all manifestations of what you thought, believed, and focused on. The good news is you can change these factors to enhance the manifestation of positive things in your life.

Practice Positive Affirmations

When you are using the Law of Attraction for weight loss, speaking out positive statements that motivate you on your goal helps you to internalize a more positive view of yourself. You can use statements like:

- I constantly lose weight every day.
- I can manage my emotions in ways that do not affect my eating patterns.
- Every day, I am changing towards my best me.
- I can do anything that I set my mind to do, and losing weight is not an exception.
- My body deserves self-love; it represents a unique part of me.
- I do not compare myself to anyone else because I cannot be anyone else, apart from myself.
- I am free from all forms of negativity that may be associated with food.
- I love and appreciate the way I look.
- My physical health is improving every day. I can feel it in my body.

Cultivate Your Brain Power

One of the important aspects of the Law of Attraction is to exercise your mind to cultivate your brainpower. Enhancing your cognitive skills improves your reasoning abilities, self-control, and positive thoughts. Here are some exercises for your mind:

- Use the hand which is not your main hand to brush your teeth. If you are left-handed, use the right hand, and if you are right-handed, use your left hand. This expands parts of the cortex that are responsible for processing information.

- Read aloud or find someone who can read anything for you while you listen. The brain takes note of various aspects of the text when it is recited than when it is read quietly.

- Take note of some tasks in your daily routines that you usually do in a particular order and switch the order you are going to complete them. This increases neural activity, while following particular routines in completing tasks decreases neural activity.

- When it's time to take your bath, take it with your eyes closed, from the time you set your feet in the shower until you have finished drying yourself. Your sensory awareness is improved by this activity.

- Engage and connect with other people during the day, more than you usually do. You can choose to talk to people over the phone or in-person rather than through text messages.

You Can Create Your Personal Reality

Thoughts are things, although you can't really see or touch them. They manifest and become your reality. It is important that you understand this and be conscious of the Law of Attraction in everything else that you are involved in, besides weight loss. Apply it in looking for the job of your dreams, personal development, on your quest for a promotion, or getting the outfit that you love. This provides you with more opportunities to witness the reality of the Law of Attraction. With time, positivity comes out more naturally, even in your efforts to lose weight.

There are considerations you should make if you want to manifest changes in your life. These are listed below:

- **Identify what you want and the reasons why:** Find out the area of your personal life you want to change. To describe the reason, find out what you do not like about your current situation in that area. For example, if it is your weight you want to change, the reason could be that you can't fit into your old, but beautiful clothes anymore.
- **Be clear on your beliefs:** What you believed before is what led you to your current situation, the one that you want to change. Your thoughts, self-talk, and actions collaboratively made you what you are now, so maintaining them will not manifest changes. You need to shift your beliefs so that they align positively with what you want. What do you think a person that needs to lose weight like you should believe about themselves? Begin to believe in that.
- **Imagine the future you:** Imagine the person that you want to be when your desired change manifests. You do not wait for it to manifest before you can see or feel how it looks like. Imagine how you are going to feel when your desired change manifests. The more you imagine it, the more your thoughts and feelings become aligned to it, and the greater the possibility of manifestation.

- **Say and behave like you have already achieved what you want:** Your self-affirmations and the way you act should be as though the changes have already manifested. Think about what a person who has what you desire does, say, and believe. Equally, think of what they would not say, do, or believe and modify your own beliefs, words, and behavior accordingly.

Believe Before Seeing

Human beings are used to seeing before believing. However, when it comes to the Law of Attraction, you need to believe before seeing. In the words of Terry Savelle-Foy, "If you can see it in your mind, you can hold it in your hands." Before you see your weight change physically, believe it, and you will see it manifesting in your life.

Chapter 7:

Mindful Eating - The Most

Important Habit for Weight Loss

Approximately 85% of overweight people who lose weight tend to regain it, or even exceed their initial weight, within a few years (Bjarnadottir, 2019). Quite often, weight gain and weight regain have been attributed to emotional eating, external eating, binge eating, and eating to appease food cravings. Extended exposure to stressful situations also promotes overeating, which often leads to obesity. It is astounding to note that people consume most of the calories that later lead to weight gain and obesity without realizing what they are "actually" doing. Progressively increasing amounts of research suggest that eating slowly and more thoughtfully can reduce weight remarkably and impacts the choices people make about the food they eat and, as well as their eating patterns. This way of eating is called mindful eating. In this chapter, you will discover how mindful eating can help you lose weight and develop a healthier relationship with food.

What Is Mindful Eating?

Mindful eating is a concept of mindfulness. It is when you pay undivided attention to the whole experience of eating and drinking (Robinson, n.d.). It involves acknowledging how you feel when you eat food, from the moment that you buy, prepare, and serve the food to the time when you place your cutlery down and clear up your dining table. Mindful eating also involves noticing all the sensations that you experience as you eat food. Your awareness of taste, satisfaction, and fullness is quite elevated when you are eating mindfully.

There is a misconception that mindful eating is about adhering to a stipulated, strict diet that forbids some types of foods. Mindful eating is also not about perfection, criticizing and appraising foods, or counting calories before or after each meal. Mindful eating does not imply that you will never give in to your cravings once in a while. It is about allowing your senses to be fully embedded in all the activities you do concerning your food, including buying or harvesting it from your garden in the backyard, cleaning it, chopping, cooking, serving the food, and eating.

Here are some recommendations on how to eat mindfully:

- Appreciate the food that you are about to eat. Connect with its appearance, taste, smell, and anything that you can note about the food.
- Don't be in a rush to eat. Eat slowly and avoid any distractions, especially visual gadgets like television. Focus on the food that you are eating.
- Find ways to cope with the guilt and anxiety that is associated with eating some types of food. Equally, learn how to cope with emotions such as stress and fear without using food.
- Learn to identify when you are really feeling hungry, and the simple quest to eat that does not necessarily sprout from hunger. While you should learn to eat in response to hunger, you should also avoid skipping meals.
- When you eat, learn to identify when you are full. It is not a matter of finishing everything that is on your plate.
- Notice how you feel when you eat. Does eating food make you feel good or sad?
- Notice how the food feels in your mouth after each bite. You can even consider putting your cutlery down after each bite to concentrate on the food in your mouth. Chew the food thoroughly and take note of how you feel as you do that.

Mindless Eating

If you are not eating mindfully, then you have been eating mindlessly. Mindless eating is the opposite of mindful eating. Are any of these mindless eating scenarios familiar to you?:

- Sitting on your couch and watching television while you are eating your food
- Eating your breakfast in the car, while driving, because you are late for work.
- Eating in your office, while your eyes are glued to your computer screen and scrolling through some items.
- The lunch hour is almost over, and you have been busy, and then you decide, "Let me just eat quickly and catch up with the meeting."
- Skipping meals and then eating to cover up all skipped meals later.
- Regard eating as a coping mechanism for stress, anxiety, or fear.
- Eating any food that is available, regardless of whether you are hungry or not, you like the food or not, let alone enjoy eating. You just eat for the sake of it.
- Overeat when you are with friends, colleagues, or some specific people in your life.

It is even easier to refrain from mindless eating when you understand the type of mindless eating that bugs you. There are different categories of mindless eaters. Take this time to analyze your eating patterns and identify the category into which you fall among the following (Albers, 2011):

- **Mindless social eating:** People who fall in this category eat more when they are in social settings and gatherings. They eat to match the way their colleagues are eating. It could be a "home scenario" where you are eating as a family, and you just can't help but eat to keep the eating pace with your spouse.

- **Mindless emotional eating:** This category has people who eat in response to emotions, good or bad emotions. They can overeat when they are excited or do the same when they are anxious.
- **Routine mindless eating:** This category describes people whose meals and eating patterns are strictly structured and inflexible. They eat at specified times, eating specific foods and specific amounts of the food, and often overlook factors such as hunger, connection with food, and satiation.
- **Multitasking mindless eating:** People in this category are used to eating while they simultaneously do something else, such as working on their computer, playing games, driving, or cooking. They tend to overeat or undereat because of the limited and divided focus on food consumption.
- **Mindless pleasure eating:** Mindless pleasure eaters react to their senses when it comes to food. Their senses tell them whether they should eat or not, and they are quite loyal to that. For example, if they smell some cookies being baked, they want to eat them as soon as the aroma reaches their noses.
- **Mindless special events eating:** As long as there are special events such as birthdays, weddings, graduation ceremonies, baby welcome parties, people in this category find themselves overeating. Usually, these people eat well on any other "normal" days with no special events.
- **Mindless night eating:** Some people do not have problems eating well as long as they can still see the sunlight. The issue comes when the sun goes down, that is when they begin to overeat. Some can even wake up in the middle of the night just to have a snack and go back to sleep.
- **Mindless eating dieting:** People in this category struggle with cravings and feeling hungry. When they decide to follow diet

rules, they sometimes feel that they are not eating enough. Sometimes, they end up eating too much in response to their cravings.

Benefits of Mindful Eating

Thich Ahat Hanh once said, "Mindful eating is very pleasant. We sit beautifully. We are aware of the people surrounding us. We are aware of the food on our plates. This is a deep practice." There is much benefit in practicing mindful eating, emotionally, socially, and physically. In this section, we will focus on the benefits that are associated with mindful eating.

It Aids Weight Loss

Reports from studies done by various researchers show *a positive link between mindful eating and healthy eating* (Ackerman, 2019, Jordan et al., 2014). It has been reported that mindful eating is associated with healthier eating patterns such as reduced consumption of calories, less impulsive, emotional, and binge eating, healthier choices of snacks and other foods. It has also been established that mindful eating shifts the preferences of individuals towards eating healthier foods. Healthier choices of foods and healthier eating patterns are both supportive of weight loss through reduced consumption of foods that cause weight gain, such as foods with excess fat.

In another study done by Jeanne Dalen and colleagues in 2010, the researchers concluded that *mindful eating could promote weight loss, improved and healthier eating behaviors, and reduction of psychological stress* in people who are obese (Dalen et al., 2010). The results from this study confirmed that mindful eating is a powerful tool in aiding weight loss. As I mentioned earlier, healthy eating habits go a long way to reducing weight and maintaining the desired weight. The stress hormone cortisol, which is released when you are under stressful conditions, can cause overeating. Here is how. Increased cortisol levels in the body also trigger the increased release of insulin, which in turn causes the sugar levels in your blood to drop. When this happens, you will begin to crave foods that are fatty and sugary. This is quite an easy way to add some pounds to your weight, but mindful eating can counter such effects of stress.

There is often some recklessness in eating when people eat outside their homes, especially when they eat in restaurants. People tend to consume more calories when they are eating in restaurants than when they eat in their homes. High-calorie food is usually sold in most restaurants, and people buy such food and eat it in large quantities. Mindful eating in restaurants was analyzed on 35 women who participated in a study done by Timmerman and Brown in 2012. The researchers in this study reported that at the end of the six weeks during which the study was done, they observed a reduction in waist circumference, weight, daily fat and calorie intake, and emotional eating in the participants. It was reported from the study that mindful eating increased diet-related self-efficacy in participants. Therefore, ***mindful eating can overcome the barriers to weight management*** that are associated with eating in restaurants.

It Treats Weight Disorders

Mindful eating can also effectively alleviate disorders that are associated with eating. In one review, an analysis was done on the effects of mindful eating interventions on binge eating. Binge eating disorders are characterized by behavioral, emotional, and physiological imbalance as far as food intake and self-identity are concerned. The study revealed that people who practice mindful eating reduced the binge eating frequency and depression symptoms that usually show up as a result of binge eating. The study also showed that mindful eating trains individuals to exercise self-control in their food choices and the frequency at which they eat (Kristeller and Wolever, 2010).

Another review, which considered 14 research articles, showed that binge eating and emotional eating could be reduced through mindfulness interventions such as mindful eating (Katterman et al., 2014). Both binge eating and emotional eating cause weight gain because they both promote overeating.

It Gives You Control Over Food

Usually, we are controlled by the food that we eat. This means that our reasons for eating, the amount of food that we eat, the time at which we eat, and the frequency at which we eat all depend on the food itself. For example, when we eat because there is an abundance of food, then we are being controlled by food availability. Similarly, when we eat large amounts of food because it tastes good, again, it is the taste of the food that determines how much we eat.

Mindful eating shifts your thoughts from making decisions based on factors around food, but based on ourselves. If you decide not to eat even when food is all over because you are not hungry, then your decision is not based on food, but on yourself. In that case, you would have exhibited control over food, and that is one of the benefits of mindful eating.

Does Eating Fast Really Matter?

Nowadays, our schedules are clogged with responsibilities at work, home, church, community societies, sports clubs, education, and other things. A single day can be so tied-up that sparing time to eat properly and slowly can sound like too much to ask. You would rather eat as fast as you can, or else you miss the appointment with a prospective employer, miss the pick-up time for your kids, lose a million-dollar contract, or miss the visitors' hour at the hospital. Despite the reasons, would you believe that eating fast is a behavior that promotes weight gain, obesity, and overeating? Yes, it is! This section explains how eating your food fast is a quick way to gain weight and increase the risk of diseases such as diabetes.

You Can Easily Overeat

To know that you are full after eating a meal, it is the brain that signals to your body that the food you have eaten is enough. However, it takes the body about 20 minutes before it can respond to the signal that is sent by the brain to tell you that you have eaten enough food. When you eat fast, there is a higher probability that you will continue to eat, and even eat too much, before you realize that you are full. By the time the brain signals are responded to by the body, you would have overeaten already. Remember, the body will not use all of the food that you would have eaten. The extra calories will lead to weight gain. Extract carbohydrates will be stored as fat, again promoting weight gain.

Eating Fast Increases the Risk of Obesity

One of the biggest health challenges that are affecting the globe is obesity. While various possible factors cause overweight and obesity, eating your food fast is one of them. A systematic review done by Ohkuma and colleagues in 2015 was aimed at determining if there was a link between the rate at which people eat food and obesity. Using information from 23 published articles, the results of the study showed a positive correlation between eating fast and increased body weight. Since a faster eating rate is associated with being overweight, it can be interpreted that it can also cause obesity.

Rapid Eating Increases the Risk of Other Health Challenges

Many other health problems are associated with eating fast, other than obesity, and being overweight. Some of these health problems are highlighted below:

- **Poor digestion:** When you eat fast, you are more likely to take bigger bites, and you might not take time to chew the food thoroughly as you should. This may affect the digestion process of the eaten food. Digestion starts in the mouth where food is mixed with digestive enzymes. When you do not chew your food properly, the food is not fully acted upon by the digestive enzymes in the saliva. Another study showed that properly chewing food also reduces calorie intake. In fact, it was reported from the same study that people who chewed their food 40 times reduced their calorie intake by 10% compared to those who chewed 15 times (Li et al., 2011). Moreover, you swallow more air when you eat your food at a too fast rate, which results in bloating and gas.
- **Insulin resistance:** Eating your food too quickly results in insulin resistance, which is characterized by surges in blood sugar and insulin concentrations. This happens when the cells in your body cannot respond to insulin and as a result, they cannot use the glucose in the blood for energy-releasing body processes. The pancreas then assumes that there is no insulin and so releases more. With time, the blood glucose levels also increase. A study by Otsuka and colleagues confirmed that eating fast is associated with insulin resistance (Otsuka et al., 2008).
- **Type 2 diabetes:** There are two causes of type 2 diabetes. It is either the pancreas does not produce insulin, or it produces the insulin, but the body fails to use it. A conclusion from one study suggested that people who eat fast have a 2.5 greater chance of getting type 2 diabetes than those that eat slowly (Radzevičienė & Ostrauskas, 2013).
- **Metabolic syndrome:** The weight gain that is caused by eating too quickly increases the likelihood of having metabolic syndrome. Metabolic syndrome is a group of conditions that occurs simultaneously, and together they increase the risk of

stroke, type 2 diabetes, and heart diseases. Some of the conditions that are included in the metabolic syndrome are excessive cholesterol, high blood sugar, and high blood pressure.

How to Eat Mindfully

Mindful meditation intends to concentrate on different aspects of the food and be aware of what happens every second as you eat. You do this using your senses of touch, taste, sound, smell, and sight, and this gives you a multidimensional experience of eating. You can learn how to eat mindfully by practicing raisin meditation.

Raisin Meditation

If you so prefer, you can do this raisin-eating experience while you read, but I would recommend that you read and understand it first, and then do it without being distracted from focusing by reading.

1. Place a small plate in front of you on a table. Now, place a raisin at the center of the plate.
2. Imagine yourself as having been just dropped from another planet to this earth. Assume that you are completely new on the earth, and there is nothing that you know about the place. Imagine that you have never experienced what it is like to be on earth, and you do not have any expectations, judgments, fears, or hopes. You just want to experience everything as it happens.
3. Look at the raisin for about 5 seconds before you pick it up.
4. Notice the weight of the raisin in your hands.
5. Examine the raisin. Remember it's your first time to see it. Look at its surface and take note of its ridges, as well as shiny and dull areas. Analyze its color.

6. Slowly bring it closer to your nose and smell it. Take note of how you react to the smell of the raisin.
7. Gently roll the raisin between your fingers, and be attentive to the sounds that it will make, if any. Observe how sticky it is on your fingers as you continue to roll it.
8. Notice how you are feeling about the raisin.
9. Now, place the raisin between your lips, and keep holding it with your fingers for about 7 seconds. Take note of what is happening within you.
10. Release the raisin from your hands into your mouth. Wait, do not chew it yet! Use your tongue to roll it in your mouth. Notice what happens to you as you do this. Take note of any taste, salivation, and any other sensations that are involved. You feel like biting it, right?
11. Take your first bite and note how that feels. Slowly chew it and allow yourself to be so embedded in the process that no sensation passes without you noticing it.
12. Don't be in a hurry to swallow. Chew the raisin until it completely liquefies in your saliva, and then swallow it.
13. As soon as you swallow, close your eyes in anticipation of the results of your experience.

Attitudes Associated With Mindful Eating

Whenever you eat mindfully, there are attitudes that should accompany your eating, should the experience bring good results of weight loss. The raisin-eating experience you learned in the previous section, must have taught you some of these attitudes if you were truly attentive to all sensations.

Don't judge: Usually, the moment you see food, judging thoughts start to come. You begin to think about whether you like the food or not, and even give yourself some reasons. You could say, "It doesn't look nice," or "The food looks great, but could it taste great too?" Do not shun your judgments off. Be aware of them because acknowledging them is an important aspect of mindful eating.

Be patient: Mindful eating requires patience because it takes much longer than rushed eating. You need to analyze the sensations involved in every step of eating, which also takes time. You take your time to chew the food, compared to what you would do with mindless eating.

Adopt the mind of a beginner: Involving your past experiences in your eating makes mindful eating more difficult. If you approach eating with the attitude of a person who is eating food for the first time, the likelihood that you will have a fuller eating experience is high. You would want to touch, smell, taste, see and listen to the food like a beginner. Besides, the same food may mean different things at different times, so it's not always a good idea to approach your present eating experience with a mindset of your past experiences with the same food.

Develop self-trust: As you become aware of the food while you eat mindfully, you develop a unique experience. This experience helps you develop self-trust based on your abilities to experience all the sensations that were embedded in your mindful eating.

Clear the "striving" mindset: With dieting, some specific parameters should be, at one point or the other, measured. With mindful eating, there are no measured parameters. In other words, there is nothing to strive for. All that you need to do is be in the present moment while you eat. Whatever happens, happens, and it's all good.

Have an accepting attitude: When you are practicing mindful eating, you need to be ready to observe, notice, and accept everything just the way you experience it. You don't need to make alterations. Float with the proceedings of the moment. For example, you may find the food tasting the way you like, while you dislike the smell. Mindful eating does not imply that you must love everything about the eating experience. You simply have to notice and accept the experience, just the way it is.

Let go of past experiences: Past experiences, observations, and expectations can negatively affect your mindful eating experience if you allow them. They will distract you from truly enjoying the experience. For example, if as a child, you resented eating raisins because you preferred chocolate. Keeping such a mindset will not allow you to have a new experience when you eat raisins.

Further Considerations for Mindful Eating

Get to know your body's hunger signals: We all have different emotional triggers that we respond to when it comes to eating. They could be frustration, stress, fear, anxiety, or loneliness, and we often listen and respond to them. However, it is best that we learn to be attentive to our body's requests for food. Check if your stomach doesn't feel light, if it is not growling, or whether you feel less energetic. How do you know that your body is hungry? These are the triggers that you should consider before deciding to eat something, rather than prioritizing your emotions.

Connect with your food: Do you often think of food regarding where it comes from, or do you perceive it as an end-product? It is quite unfortunate that most of us have lost touch with the journey that food travels before it becomes a meal on our plates. Consider the water, air, and soil that contributed to food growth, the farmers who did the planting, maintenance, and harvesting. Consider the people who brought the food from the farms to the shops where it was repackaged, those who arranged it on the shelves in an attractive manner, and "you" who bought and prepared the food. These are just some of the hands through which the food passed; there should be more contributions that were made to make the food a nutritional meal that you are delighted to eat and satiate yourself. When you think about your food in this manner, you will learn to be grateful for it. You will feel the connection between you, the food, the people you are eating with, the people who made all efforts to make the food available, and the universe that provided the important elements that help plants and animals grow.

Let your body collaborate with your brain: Normally, the body sends signals that you have eaten enough 20 minutes after the brain has signaled the same thing. Therefore, when you eat quickly, you do give your body enough time to catch up with the brain's signals, and you will continue to eat without realizing that you are overeating. If you eat slowly, you give your body and mind enough time to collaborate so that you can feel it when you are satiated. Easier ways to ensure that you eat slowly are by giving yourself enough time to chew your food, swallowing your food before adding more into your mouth, and putting down your cutlery between mouthfuls. Eat more slowly so that you can listen to the signals that are sent by your body.

Create a mindful kitchen: Have you ever noticed that the meals that we eat alone are more random compared to those that we eat with others, be it they are friends, colleagues, or family? Rather than searching through your kitchen cupboards for what you can eat, make meals that you eat at a consistent time and in an organized manner too. Choose to put your food on plates, sit at the dining table, use cutlery instead of your hands, and eat together with others. Eating with others also helps you eat slowly, as you converse with others, between mouthfuls, of course.

Avoid distractions: You eat more mindfully when you eat without distractions. Eating while watching the television or your computer screen are mindless eating habits that often lead to overeating. Take note of the situations where you eat while you are surrounded by distractions to strategize on how best you can avoid such situations. For example, if you usually eat your breakfast while driving to work because you are always late, try to wake up a bit earlier, prepare your breakfast, and eat at home before you leave for work.

The two-plate approach: This approach is appropriate in places where it is difficult or impossible for you to control your portion size, such as at a party with a buffet. Take two plates, one of which should be smaller, and this will be your eating plate. The other one will be your serving plate. Put all the food that you think you might eat on the serving plate. Once you sit down, take food from the serving plate and put it on your eating plate. Eat your food in a slow, mindful way, taking note of your body's signals so that you do not overeat. When you finish the food that is on your eating plate, listen to your body. If it is satiated, stop eating, but if not, take another portion from your serving plate and place it on your eating plate and eat as you did for the previous portion.

Mindful eating plate: This is when the standard dinner plate is divided into four sections. The first section represents *observation*, where you take note of your body, whether you are hungry, satiated, energetic or not, or rumbling. The other section represents *savoring*, where you focus on the texture, aroma, flavor, and taste of the food. The third section represents *"being in the present moment,"* and here you do everything that makes you focus on eating. For example, sit down, switch off the television, and just eat. The fourth section reminds you to be *non-judging*. Avoid thoughts that make you feel guilty. A glass of water would represent *appreciation* to all the people who contributed to produce the food.

Eat with your non-dominant hand: When you eat with your non-dominant hand, you eat fewer calories. Research shows that people who eat with their non-dominant hand consume 30% less food than when they eat with their dominant hand (Benshosan, 2020).

Strategize on how to reduce portion sizes: Some things in our homes determine the portion size of our food. Imagine placing the same portion size of food in a bigger and smaller plate. By just looking at the plates, it looks like the portion in the bigger plate is smaller.

Remember, the size of the portions is the same! Therefore, if you serve your food on a bigger plate, there is a greater probability that you will feel less satiated, or even ask for more, while you would have felt satiated if you had eaten from a smaller plate. You can consider using salad plates for your food portions, rather than the standard dinner plates.

Conclusion

The challenge that most people face is not just how to lose weight, but how to lose it and maintain their desired weight once it has been reached. Most diets and exercise regimes successfully reduce weight for some time, and sometimes, the targeted weight loss is even reached. However, the frustrations come when people regain the weight that they would have lost or even more than it.

This book revealed the special secret that most diet plans and exercise regimes lack, which helps you shed those extra pounds and maintain your desired weight. Most diets and exercise regimes focus on the external factors of weight loss, which are outside an individual. The motivation that comes from outside an individual is usually short-lived and difficult to maintain. You are forced to shift your lifestyle. Well, if you have tried them before, you will agree with me that you can only endure a drift from your normal lifestyle for a while, but sooner or later, you get tired and get back to your old way of doing things.

Weight-loss tools that are introduced in this book focus on the inner being. They target the root cause of unhealthy behaviors and modify them from within. Behaviors do not emanate from outside a person, but from within, which is the more reason why weight loss methods such as hypnosis, meditation, mindful eating, practicing positivity, and appropriate motivation have been brought forward. When weight loss is targeted from within an individual, it becomes less regarded as a goal but as one of the benefits of leading a healthy life. Lifetime good health becomes the main goal, but you still lose weight anyway. The best part is you can maintain the body that you want way after you reach your target weight, or even for a lifetime, because healthy eating behaviors will become a norm than an obligation as time goes on.

All behaviors are embedded in your subconscious mind. Therefore, weight loss tools such as hypnosis help you access the subconscious mind and reprogram it to adopt new behaviors by suggesting what you want to do. It's a learning process for the mind that does not happen in a single click, but it surely brings positive results in the long run. Together with meditation, hypnosis also alleviates factors such as stress, which are associated with weight gain. Stress hormones such as cortisol which are released when you are exposed to stressful situations, increase carbohydrate and fat metabolism in the body to release quick energy. This increases the secretion of insulin, leading to the depletion of blood sugar levels. When blood sugar levels deplete, your appetite and cravings for sugary, fatty, and salty foods increases.

Mindful eating has a special role in long-term weight loss. It involves allowing all your senses to be part of the eating process while you focus on what is happening in the present moment, as far as eating is concerned. You become extremely aware of the aroma, taste, appearance, sounds, and texture of the food that you eat. Mindful eating not only focuses on the eating process but also on all the steps that occur before the food becomes a meal on your plate. This includes what happens at the farm where crops are grown and animals are reared until you buy, prepare, and eat the food. This helps you be grateful for the food you eat, developing a positive relationship with food that ultimately helps you make the right food choices.

Weight loss also depends on what we think and how we speak about ourselves, and what we desire in our lives. The Law of Attraction states that "like attracts like." If you think and speak positively, your body vibrates at a certain frequency, and the things that align to the frequency at which you vibrate are attracted into your life. The same thing happens when you think and speak negative affirmations about yourself. Therefore, if you desire to lose weight, think about it, believe it before it happens, and say it out loud with positivity. Behave the way that you would if you had lost the weight already. Tell yourself, "It is time to really lose weight and maintain my new body!"

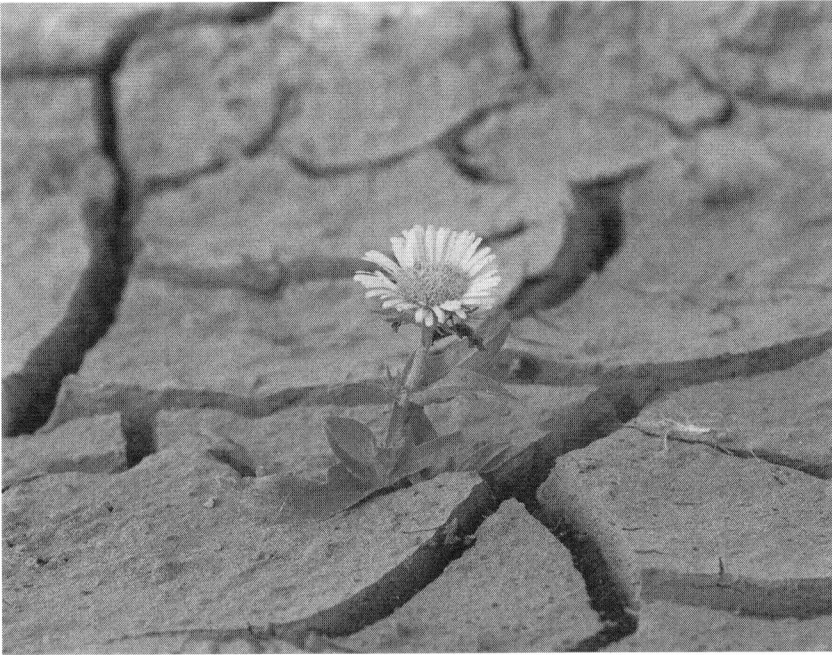

Figure 3: Positivity is key.

If you can use the tools that are provided in this book, positivity will be written all over you, from the way you think, eat, talk, behave, and motivate yourself. Go out there and use them to lose weight, and even beyond that, live your life the best and positive way. Again, if you enjoyed this book, please leave a review on Amazon.

Self-Worth Affirmations

❖ I am unique. I feel good about being alive and being me.

❖ Life is fun and rewarding.

❖ Amazing opportunities exist for me in every aspect of my life.

❖ There are no such things as problems, only opportunities.

❖ I love challenges; they bring out the best in me.

❖ I replace "I must", "I should" and "I have to" with "I choose". (try it with something you think you have to do, and replace must with choose... notice the difference?)

❖ I choose to be happy right now. I love my life.

❖ I appreciate everything I have. I live in joy.

❖ I am courageous. I am willing to act in spite of any fear.

❖ I am positive and optimistic. I believe things will always work out for the best.

❖ It's easy to make friends. I attract positive and kind people into my life.

❖ It's easy to meet people. I create positive and supportive relationships.

❖ I am a powerful creator. I create the life I want.

❖ I am OK as I am. I accept and love myself.

❖ I am confident. I trust myself.

❖ I am successful right now.

❖ I am passionate. I am outrageously enthusiastic and inspire others.

- ❖ I am calm and peaceful.

- ❖ I have unlimited power at my disposal.

- ❖ I am optimistic. I believe things will always work out for the best.

- ❖ I am kind and loving. I am compassionate and truly care for others.

- ❖ I am focused and persistent. I will never quit.

- ❖ I am energetic and enthusiastic. Confidence is my second nature.

- ❖ I treat everyone with kindness and respect.

- ❖ I inhale confidence and exhale fear.

- ❖ I am flexible. I adapt to change quickly.

- ❖ I have integrity. I am totally reliable. I do what I say.

- ❖ I am competent, smart and able.

- ❖ I believe in myself,

- ❖ I recognize the many good qualities I have.

- ❖ I see the best in other people.

- ❖ I surround myself with people who bring out the best in me.

- ❖ I let go of negative thoughts and feelings about myself.

- ❖ I love who I have become.

- ❖ I am always growing and developing.

- ❖ My opinions resonate with who I am.

- ❖ I am congruent in everything I say and do.

- ❖ I deserve to be happy and successful

- ❖ I have the power to change myself

- ❖ I can forgive and understand others and their motives

- ❖ I can make my own choices and decisions

- ❖ I am free to choose to live as I wish and to give priority to my desires

- ❖ I can choose happiness whenever I wish no matter what my circumstances

- ❖ I am flexible and open to change in every aspect of my life

- ❖ I act with confidence having a general plan and accept plans are open to alteration

- ❖ It is enough to have done my best

- ❖ I deserve to be loved

- ❖ I have high self-esteem

- ❖ I love and respect myself.

- ❖ I am a great person.

- ❖ I respect myself deeply.

- ❖ My thoughts and opinions are valuable.

- ❖ I am confident that I can achieve anything.

- ❖ I have something special to offer the world.

- ❖ Others like and respect me.

- ❖ I am a wonderful human being I feel great about myself and my life.

- ❖ I am worthy of having high self-esteem.

- ❖ I believe in myself.

- ❖ I deserve to feel good about myself.

- ❖ I know I can achieve anything.

- ❖ Having respect for myself helps others to like and respect me.

- ❖ Feeling good about myself is normal for me.

- ❖ Improving my self-esteem is very important.

- ❖ Being confident in myself comes naturally to me.

- ❖ Liking and respecting myself is easy.

- ❖ Speaking my mind with confidence is something I just naturally do.

- ❖ Each day I notice I am more self-discipline.

- ❖ I enjoy being self-disciplined.

❖ I am doing the best I can with the knowledge and experience I have obtained so far.

❖ It's OK to make mistakes. They are opportunities to learn.

❖ I always follow through on my promises.

❖ I treat others with kindness and respect.

❖ I see myself with kind eyes.

❖ I am a unique and a very special person.

❖ I love myself more each day.

❖ I am willing to change.

❖ I approve of myself.

❖ I care about myself.

- ❖ I am a child of God.

- ❖ My work gives me pleasure.

- ❖ I give praise freely.

- ❖ I am respected by others.

- ❖ I rejoice in my uniqueness.

- ❖ I attract praise.

- ❖ I deserve good in my life.

- ❖ I appreciate myself.

- ❖ Each day I am becoming more self-confident.

Download the AUDIOBOOK Version

of This Book for FREE

Follow the QR Codes Below to GET STARTED!

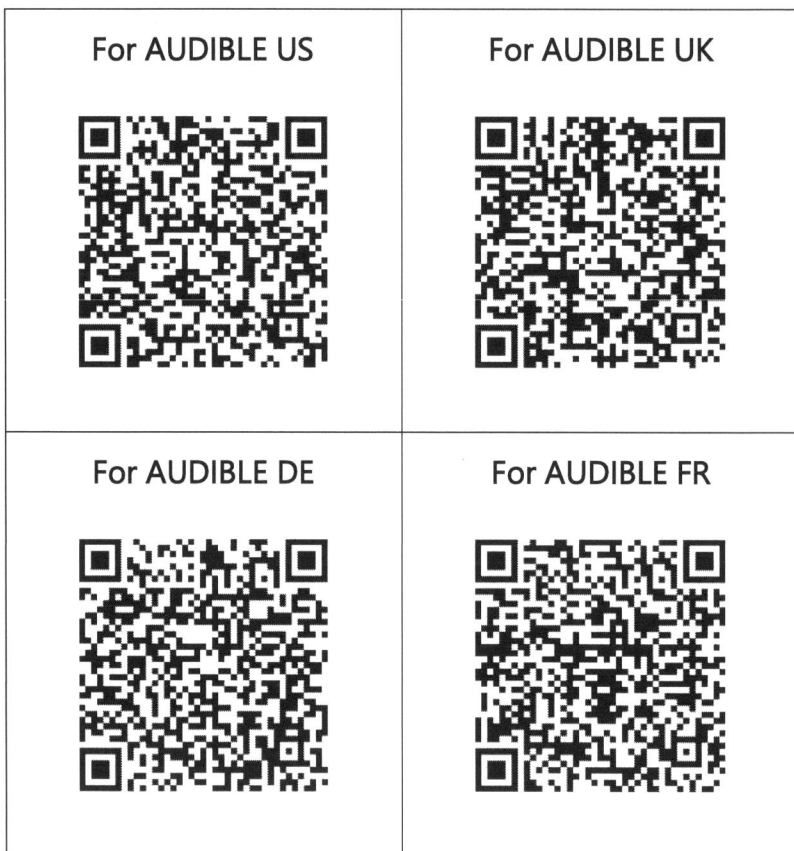

For AUDIBLE US	For AUDIBLE UK
For AUDIBLE DE	For AUDIBLE FR

★★★

I Would Really Appreciate It If You Left a Review, It's Very Important.

★★★

Made in the USA
Monee, IL
01 March 2021